ULRIKA DAVIDSSON
RAW FOOD
DETOX

Over 100 Recipes for Better Health, Weight Loss, and Increased Vitality

Photography by Malte Danielsson

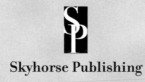

Skyhorse Publishing

Skyhorse Publishing books may be purchased in bulk at special
discounts for sales promotion, corporate gifts, fund-raising, or
educational purposes. Special editions can also be created to
specifications. For details, contact the Special Sales Department,
Skyhorse Publishing, 307 West 36th Street, 11th Floor, New York, NY
10018 or info@skyhorsepublishing.com.

Skyhorse® and Skyhorse Publishing® are registered trademarks of
Skyhorse Publishing, Inc.®, a Delaware corporation.

Visit our website at www.skyhorsepublishing.com

Translation by Stine Osttveit

10 9 8 7 6 5 4 3 2 1

Library of Congress Cataloging-in-Publication Data is available on
file.

ISBN: 978-1-61608-626-8

Printed in China

CONTENTS

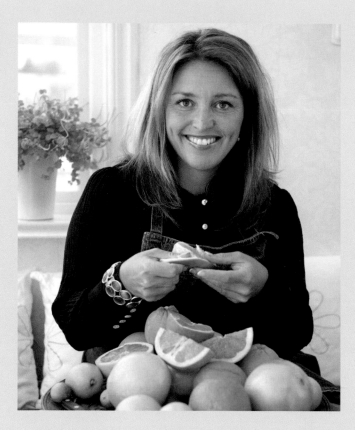

A NEW, CLEANER WORLD

I am a typical mother of two: married for fifteen years, living in a two-story house outside of Stockholm, working almost full-time with a husband that works overtime. Every day basically looks the same: I wake up my family, eat a quick breakfast, get everyone out the door to school or work, work all day with a quick break for lunch, go grocery shopping on my way home, make dinner, do dishes, drive my children to their afterschool activities, tidy up, then finally end up exhausted in front of the TV around 9:00 PM.

Does this sound familiar to anyone?

In 2005 I decided to become a nutritionist after I successfully lost about seventy pounds by sticking to the GI (Glycemic Index) Diet. I was fascinated by the importance of diet and food choices and I changed my own eating habits dramatically. Since then, I have been working full-time writing GI nutritional books as well as articles and recipes for multiple publications. I've held seminars and classes on both the GI and LCHF (Low Carb High Fat) regimen that have been attended by thousands of people, and I am currently recognized as one of Sweden's leading nutritionists.

Through my work, I've come across numerous individuals (mostly women) who just generally don't feel well. Usually they suffer from headaches, joint pains, lack of sleep, poor metabolism, and fatigue. Many of them also struggle with another problem: They can't lose weight, despite their battles with various diets.

For the last three years I have worked largely with detox and cleansing, and I am now enjoying the results. I would claim that detoxifying and raw food provide one thing that any other diet would not accomplish nearly as well—namely, boosting energy. The fact that raw food and detox will also make you look and feel younger, thinner, and healthier all around is an added bonus.

Even nutritional experts are in a constant state of evolution, and since my last book, *Lose Weight and Cleanse the Body with Detox* (2008), I have learned even more about both cleansing and raw food. It is this knowledge that I would like to share with you here. I hope that you will take joy in my new discoveries, as well as, of course, all the energy-boosting recipes and mouthwatering and motivating pictures that you will find in this book.

Enjoy!

Ulrika

A TYPICAL DAY: 4:45 PM

It's time for the woman of the household to decide on a dinner for the evening. Despite all the progress we've made and debates about gender equality, a recently released study shows that this is still the woman's responsibility. That the decision of what to serve is usually not planned out, but rather is rushed, will most often result in the choice of something quick and easy because we just don't have time for anything else.

Some of the most common dinner choices in the U.S. are spaghetti, pizza, breaded or fried meats with instant mashed potatoes, macaroni and cheese, and tacos.

WE CONSUME

- Large quantities of refined sugars
- A cocktail of flavor enhancers, food coloring, pesticides, and preservatives
- Chemically treated trans fats that are added to foods so that they will keep
- Factory-produced milk that undergoes a variety of processes before reaching store shelves
- An average of 634 cups (150 liters) of coffee per person per year
- 40 cups (9.4 liters) of pure alcohol per person per year

SUGAR

The amount of sugar in our food has been rising steadily since the '70s. It has gotten to the point where we have become accustomed to a sweet taste in almost all the foods we eat. Ham, sausage, bread, sauces, yogurt, and cereals are all examples of daily foods that contain added sugar. You may not have thought about the fact that sugar is an ingredient in these products. As we have come to buy and eat preprepared foods in greater quantities, we have lost control of the amount of sugar we consume.

One of the main reasons why sugar has become a common ingredient in our food is the ever-increasing demand for low-fat and low-calorie products. Sugar has taken the place of fat as a natural flavor enhancer. Is sugar better for you than fat? Most certainly not. Have we really been deceived all these years?

Unfortunately, the answer is yes, and today we are clearly experiencing the repercussions. The obesity epidemic is more severe than ever before, and the number of people diagnosed with type 2 diabetes has increased dramatically.

We have also been tricked into choosing sweeteners in place of natural sugar and have adopted the misconceived notion that consuming diet sodas, sugar-free gum, and sugar-free candy is a healthy alternative to the real thing. The reality is that these products are one of our bodies' worst enemies. Today we know that many sweeteners affect our bodies negatively, although we have yet to see the final consequences of our consumption. Artificial sweeteners are chemically produced sugars that alter our feelings of hunger, our brain, and our nervous system. Recently, researchers have found that artificial sweeteners are one of the causes of the growing obesity problem. And this may just be the tip of the iceberg, as we have yet to discover the extent of the negative effects sweeteners may have on our bodies, which could include intestinal problems, allergies, and inflammation.

ADDITIVES

The amount of poison in our foods has increased dramatically since the '60s. Do you think that it's natural for our foods to be sprayed and packed with food coloring, stabilizers, preservatives, chemically produced additives, and trans fats? It's impossible for the body to properly break many of these things down, leading to an imbalance in the body that may make you sick.

Modern food is very different from the food of previous generations; it is therefore that much more important that you stay informed so that you can make the right food choices and avoid dangerous additives. The lower the percentage of natural ingredients the greater the percentage of other ingredients such as water, potato flour, milk powder, trans fats, sugars, and other cheap junk your food is likely to contain. The fact that additives are approved does not necessarily mean that they are good for your health. Ideally, you should always choose organic and additive-free foods.

TRANS FATS

Trans fat is an unnatural fat produced when cheap vegetable oils are chemically treated to create a fluid consistency and a long shelf life. This kind of fat builds up in your body because it cannot be properly broken down. Trans fats increase the level of dangerous LDL cholesterol (low density lipoprotein) in the body while decreasing the good HDL cholesterol (high density lipoprotein). In addition, it raises your triglyceride levels, which increases the risk of deadly heart and artery disease.

Trans fats are most commonly found in ready-to-eat baked goods (including certain breads), frozen dinners, ice cream, sauces, and instant mashed potatoes. The best way to avoid trans fat is to carefully read the label of everything you buy.

MILK

We've all grown up believing that milk is good for you, and many families name milk as their healthy drink of choice because they think that it is a natural product that supports our body's well-being.

But the milk we consume is a far cry from the milk that is initially extracted from dairy cows. By the time you pour that milk into your glass it's been regulated, pasteurized, homogenized, and infused with added vitamins, and has lost much of its taste, nutrition value, and enzymes in the process.

Today's research shows that milk can be harmful and may contribute to gastrointestinal problems as well as allergies and inflammation.

ALCOHOL

The consumption of alcohol is steadily increasing, and we tend to drink alcohol more often and in larger quantities than in the past. Wine, cocktails, and beer are served at most social gatherings, and it is more common than ever to uncork a bottle of wine at the end of a long day, weekday or not. Many use wine to unwind after a stressful day at work, and once the bottle is open we often end up pouring a glass to top off a regular Monday, Tuesday, or any day we think that we deserve a special little treat.

Many experience headaches as a side effect of wine—especially red wine—and the truth is that when we really start looking at what wine contains, the facts are alarming. In order to keep pests and bacteria from disturbing the grapes, cultivators will spray them with chemicals to prevent mold, among other things. Today there are no set policies regulating what wineries can add to wine during production, and many wineries will add chemical substances as general protocol just to avoid the possibility of unwanted bacteria.

COFFEE

Coffee is one of the world's most pesticide treated and processed foodstuffs. The effects of this on both the environment and our health are disturbing. The pesticides used are poisonous, and people can die from exposure to them. The soil is exhausted by the extremely large-scale and repetitive growing of crops, and watercourses are ruined by the discharge from the pesticides. Highly poisonous pesticides are used on 70 percent of crops. In Costa Rica alone, 700 cases of acute poisoning are reported each year, and each year thirty people die as a result. In Brazil harm resulting from exposure to pesticides is the largest health risk in the country, and it is believed that approximately 200,000 people are affected by these toxins. Toxin exposure also affects the individuals who work with the spraying of pesticides, more often than not without adequate protective gear.

DRUGS

If we're not feeling well we go to the doctor and get a prescription for medication. Over the course of the last forty years, the use of medications and drugs has increased at a staggering rate. Is our good health increasing as well? Unfortunately not. Instead of trying to locate the underlying causes of our headaches, heart and artery disease, diabetes, gastrointestinal problems, rheumatism, and so forth, we opt for the quick and easy relief of drugs. Popping painkillers every day, taking penicillin, and asking the doctor for cholesterol reducers are quick fixes that don't require any real commitment to addressing the underlying causes of these problems. A better approach would be to identify the real issue and allow the body to heal itself through a healthy diet, detoxifying, rest, and exercise.

ENVIRONMENTAL TOXINS AND CHEMICALS

During a regular morning routine, we typically come into contact with thirty to forty different kinds of chemicals. First, we shower with shampoo and conditioner. We wash our bodies with soap, and after drying off we apply lotion and deodorant. To our face we then apply a day cream, foundation, rouge, mascara, and eye shadow. After brushing our teeth with toothpaste, we apply lip gloss and top it all off with a few spritzes of perfume. Lastly, we'll style our hair with mousse and hairspray. Put it all together and you have a fairly normal morning routine for women and girls.

Every single day we are exposed to tens of thousands of chemicals that were virtually nonexistent on our planet just decades ago. Today, every human being is affected by chemicals one way or the other. In the '40s, we utilized approximately one million tons of chemicals; today, that number has increased to a staggering 500,000 million tons yearly. Needless to say, this is the world's fastest growing industry.

The uninhibited spread of chemicals has become one of our most serious environmental issues. Although research on the subject is still limited, a growing number of people are becoming aware of the grave health risks exposure to these toxins and chemicals can lead to. Osteoporosis, diabetes, allergies, reproductive problems, and cancer are only a few examples of the many afflictions that research has traced to environmental toxins and chemicals.

INCREASED EXPOSURE TO DANGEROUS SUBSTANCES

We live in a time in which more and more toxins are gradually sneaking into our daily lives. Our body will work to cleanse itself of toxins naturally; however, there is a limit to our body's capacity to do this. When the strain is too much for the body to handle, we become ill. We feel tired, we have headaches, rashes, allergies, and soreness, and our immune system suffers. Our body's natural detoxification utilizes nutrients in the form of vitamins, minerals, and amino acids. If our bodies are lacking in these key nutrients, the detoxification process shuts down, and we end up storing these toxins in our bodies.

A good way to restore the body's balance and prevent illness is to take the time to consider your eating habits and your daily (often) bad food choices. There are so many good and healthy foods to eat and tasty recipes to prepare. Don't get stuck with the wrong habits; take a step toward improving your health. I will be so bold as to guarantee that you will feel better than ever before.

THE THEORY BEHIND RAW FOOD

All animals and living beings, with the exception of humans, live off of a 100 percent raw diet—and who is getting sicker as a result of the foods they consume? None other than us humans.

"Raw food" is a term used to describe food that is not cooked at temperatures over 107 degrees (42 C). This method of cooking allows important nutrients as well as enzymes—which help your metabolism—to stay in the food we eat. When we cook food at high temperatures many of the important nutrients disappear, and harmful toxins are released instead.

If you're suffering from bad health, the benefits of following the raw food regimen are vast. Many find that their bodies function better, with an improved metabolism, increased energy, and greater mental balance. The purer the foods you eat, the easier it becomes to understand your body's signals.

BACK TO NATURE

The interest in raw and nutritious food is growing by the minute, and the demand for natural, quality ingredients and organic foods is stronger than ever. The additives, chemicals, and high temperatures we use to prepare our meals are ruining the food's natural nutritional value. Many are under the misconception that "raw food" refers only to raw vegetables and fresh fruit, when in reality there is much more to it than that. Keeping a strict diet based on fresh fruit and vegetables alone may become very challenging, and you do not necessarily have to follow the raw food diet 100 percent of the time to reap some of its benefits. You will experience a significant difference just by altering some of your regular food choices. The purpose of raw food is to keep your body healthy and to gain energy. A diet that consists of about 75 percent raw food is a good goal, but even if you just want to make one meal a week raw food that is still better than nothing—you just need to find a balance that suits you.

The raw food diet has been practiced all over the world for quite some time with remarkable results. Today you can find many different approaches to raw food; some approaches will allow dairy and meats while others are based on a strict vegan diet that consists entirely of vegetables, fruits, sprouts, nuts, seeds, algae, cold-pressed vegetable oils, spices, and honey.

My recipes are based on a vegan diet, but with the addition of boiled legumes, rice, quinoa, and roasted root vegetables, along with goat and sheep cheeses. About 75 percent of the book's recipes are based on a strict raw food regimen; however, some dishes are prepared at temperatures over 107 degrees (42 C). The reason why I boil, bake, and roast at higher temperatures is simply that the results are not as good at lower temperatures. Also, it's just very difficult to achieve the results that I want.

WHY ENZYMES ARE IMPORTANT FOR THE BODY

Enzymes naturally exist in all foods, but they are partly eliminated during high-temperature cooking. That is why raw vegetables and fruits are so important for our bodies.

We do produce our own enzymes, but as we grow older our natural production slows down and this affects our health negatively. Alcohol, stress, and toxins will slow production down even more. It is not surprising then that the level of enzymes is low in most middle-aged men and women. Many health experts claim that because of the low level of enzymes that exist in our bodies and our failure to replenish them through our diets we also age faster.

When we eat raw food, which has a high enzyme content capable of refilling our depositories, it is not necessary to rely on our own energy as much as we would on a different diet. I am sure you have experienced a "food coma" after a heavy meal once or twice. With raw food this will disappear, because the food you eat is easily digestible and will give—rather than consume—energy. Enzymes assist the digestive process and contribute to the healthy gastrointestinal floras that we need to stay healthy, energized, and strong. Good health will also strengthen your immune system.

PREPARING RAW FOOD

Choose organic ingredients because they contain more nutrients and fewer toxins. Many conventional growers will use chemicals and GMOs (genetically modified organisms). This is done to increase the size of the crop, speed up the growing process, and fight pests and bacteria. Organic crops are only enhanced through the addition of minerals, and the crops mature at a natural pace, which makes them higher in vitamins and minerals.

The raw food regimen is mostly vegetarian. It is also common to avoid dairy and wheat because they are usually both heated and processed. As an alternative you can use buckwheat flour, coconut flour, and rice flour. Buy oat milk or make your own by mixing oats with a little bit of water. Regular white sugar is substituted with honey, agave syrup, dried fruit, fresh berries, or fruits.

Avoid cooking food at high temperatures as much as possible. You can lightly heat vegetables using a wok, or steam ingredients that need that extra heat for preparation. Some of the soups in this book are boiled and are therefore not proper raw food; however, they are still high in necessary nutrients. The same goes for some of my other recipes; I bake the bread in the oven and boil the quinoa, but for most of the dishes a light heating below 107 degrees (42 C) is all that is needed. By mixing, drying, and marinating the ingredients you can make everything from smoothies and soups to ice cream, pizza, pies, and candy.

You may also create variations on the different dishes by changing the spices and herbs. In some of the recipes I use nonraw food ingredients such as coconut milk, ajvar (a Serbian relish made from red bell peppers, eggplant, garlic, and chili pepper), canned tomatoes, preprepared pesto, and bouillon. I do this either to save time or for a lack of better alternatives.

In your kitchen you should have a dehydrator (for cooking at temperatures below 200 degrees), a food processor, a blender, and, if possible, a juicer. Aside from these a regular oven, a sauce pan, and a frying pan will be more than enough to prepare these recipes.

IS RAW FOOD FOR EVERYONE?

Anyone can try a raw food diet. Just remember that the first couple of days you may feel different, and you may miss certain foods that you are used to consuming significant amounts of, such as bread and milk. Once you start getting into the routine of eating raw and discover the diverse array of tasty foods you can choose from, you will start making new and better food choices. You may attempt to get the whole family to try raw food—if you do not wish to follow the strict vegetarian regimen, you may supplement it with fish, seafood, eggs, or white or red meats.

THE THEORY BEHIND DETOX

During the five years I have been working with the practice of detoxifying as a professional nutritionist, I have seen amazing results. I highly recommend detoxifying two to three times a year in order to cleanse the body and get rid of stored toxins and waste.

After two weeks of detoxifying, your organs will begin to function better and you will easily sense what kinds of foods the body responds positively to and the foods you should be avoiding. If you've been struggling with soreness, gastrointestinal problems, lack of sleep, etc., and you feel better after the detox, you should evaluate your eating habits and try to introduce as much raw food as you possibly can. If you have the desire and the opportunity to continue the detox at the end of the two weeks you may absolutely do so. For many people the detox experience changes everything, leaving them feeling better than they ever have before.

CTRL+ALT+DELETE

You can compare the detox to pressing ctrl+alt+delete on your computer's keyboard. When your computer freezes you press these three buttons to get it to restart. This is exactly what a detox does for your body—the body is cleansed and revitalized, and emerges with newfound strength.

If you have any of these symptoms, then a detox will help you to feel better:

- You have trouble losing weight
- You are always tired and have trouble sleeping
- You are constipated or have other gastrointestinal issues
- You suffer from digestive problems
- You regularly experience soreness in joints or muscles (Rheumatism or Fibromyalgia)
- You suffer from rashes or allergies
- You have dry skin or a problem with itching
- You frequently suffer from headaches
- You sweat more than normal
- You suffer from bad breath
- You suffer from stress
- You have mood swings
- You feel depressed

TEN REASONS TO DO A DETOX

1. Weight loss – You will most likely lose weight and your vital signs will improve. It is normal to lose about 4–6 pounds the first ten days.

2. More energy – When you get rid of all of the toxins and other waste products in your body your energy level will significantly increase. After five or six days it's common to feel like the time is just flying by, and your energy levels will be stable from morning until late at night.

3. Improved digestion – Even if you do not feel like you're struggling with your digestion now, you will experience a difference. Issues like bloating, acid reflux, and irregular bowel movements will disappear.

4. Sleeping better – Many find that they sleep more soundly and are generally more relaxed and balanced. The main reason for this is that you are not consuming alcohol or coffee.

5. Allergies and rashes – While these will not go completely away, they will get better. Breakouts are often relieved and if you have an allergy, to pollen for example, the detox will make it easier for your body to cope with it.

6. Strong immune system – The detox promotes an alkaline intestinal flora, and you also eat a large amount of antioxidants and vitamins that will strengthen your immune system as well as your whole body.

7. Balance – This is something you have to experience firsthand! Through the process of detoxifying the body achieves an inner harmony and balance that noticeably improves your general well-being.

8. Better skin – Your skin will glow, and acne and other breakouts will diminish or disappear completely. Tendencies to get stretch marks will decrease and many say that they experience firmer skin.

9. Shiny hair – You will experience a great difference in the quality of your hair. After a few weeks you will be able to see and feel that it is thicker, shinier, and more full of life.

10. A longer life – A diet rich in vitamins, antioxidants, minerals, and healthy fats strengthens all of the body's organs. If you also continue to decrease your intake of toxins, such as coffee, drugs, salt, additives, and pesticides, chances are that you will live a longer life.

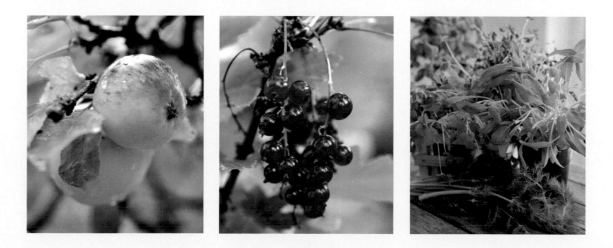

13

THE TWO-WEEK DETOX

Plan your detox carefully. You should stick to the regimen for at least two weeks in order to achieve noticeable and long-lasting effects. During the first few days the body will break down and clear out waste, which means that there will be so-called free radicals circulating. You may therefore feel sluggish and experience some bodily discomfort and drowsiness. After four to five days these symptoms will subside and you will begin to experience the aforementioned surge of energy.

HOW MUCH SHOULD YOU EAT?

You will be cutting down on the volume of food you eat, but you will still feel satisfied with the quantities you are consuming. Mostly, you will be eating natural carbohydrates, natural fats, and a relatively small quantity of protein. The reason for this is that the liver needs to be working on breaking down toxins and waste, and should not have to break down proteins, which consumes additional energy.

EXAMPLE OF A REGULAR DAY ON THE DETOX

Breakfast (7:30 AM)
A glass of water with a spritz of lemon
Soy yogurt with fresh fruit, berries, and nuts
A cup of tea

Snack (10:00 AM)
Almond muffins with apples and cinnamon and a cup of tea

Lunch (12:00 PM)
Cauliflower tabouleh with halloumi and mint guacamole

Afternoon snack (3:00 PM)
Pineapple and mango smoothie

Dinner (07:00 PM)
Beet quinoa with pea pesto

THE TRANSITIONAL PHASE

1. Begin your detox at the end of the week, on a Thursday for example. This way you will have the weekend to rest and take it easy. The drowsiness usually disappears after a few days, so you will be ready for work again on Monday.

2. You may follow the detox regimen for up to four weeks. After that you should start introducing other foods again. After four weeks you may start introducing proteins, both animal- and vegetable-based, or you may choose to continue eating strictly vegetarian.

DETOX AND EXERCISE

Detox weeks are not a good time to be training for a marathon, but rather a time to allow the body to rest. Avoid the gym, intense spinning classes, and other forms of high-intensity exercise. Try going for a walk or a bike ride instead, or you can turn to yoga or Pilates. Listen to your body and do not push it too hard.

ORGANIC

Choose organic vegetables and fruits whenever possible. You should make this a general rule, to be followed not only while you are detoxing, but always.

SUPPLEMENTS

You can complete the detox without supplements; however, I do recommend taking them to give your body a boost. Choose supplements according to quality and not to price; sometimes the most expensive brand is also the most effective.

Personally, I use First Cleanse or Pure Cleanse from ReNew Life, Ultra Clear plus from Alpha-Plus, and Ultra detox from Holistics. All of these products contain cleansing herbs and other plants that aid the body in breaking down toxins and waste.

• You should also take probiotics for a healthy intestinal flora. You can easily buy this at any drugstore. I also recommend taking probiotics following any antibiotics treatment.

• If you tend to suffer from digestive problems you may also take digestive enzymes. One capsule taken with larger meals will make you feel a lot better after you've eaten.

• Fibers are also very important because they absorb toxins and waste and help you expel these through bowel movements. The brands I previously mentioned all contain fiber from either oats or psyllium husk.

• Other supplements that aid digestion include super-berry powders like açai and blueberry, and so-called greens such as spirulina, algae, chlorella, buckthorn, wheatgrass, rosehips, and plant extracts. Blend these with water and drink them every day for a cleansing effect.

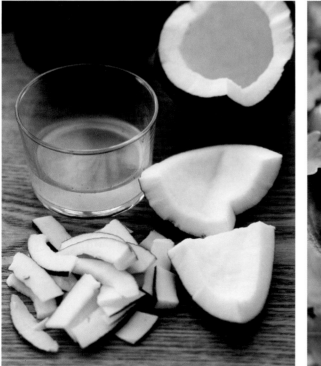
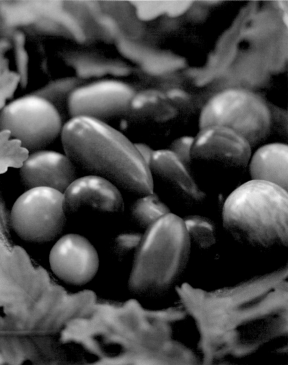

EAT OFTEN

Fats: Cold-pressed olive oil, canola oil, and selected other vegetable oils are okay, but avoid cheap versions. Choose a high-quality oil and shy away from hydrogenated oils. You may also buy coconut oil; this is a stable fat, which is excellent for cooking and baking. You should use coconut milk in your sauces, but avoid the low-fat versions.

• Nuts and seeds of all kinds are fine; just remember that they should be unsalted. You may roast them yourself in a dry skillet and add spices and salt to your liking. This is an easy way to avoid hydrogenated fat, which is commonly found in salted nuts. Make sure you vary the kinds of nuts you eat. Rather than just eating peanuts or cashews, you may also try almonds, walnuts, hazelnuts, and Brazil nuts.

• Pumpkin seeds, flaxseeds, sesame seeds, and sunflower seeds make good toppings for yogurt, or they may also be used in home-baked breads and crackers.

• Avocado is a great source of fat. Use it to make guacamole that you can dip your vegetables in, or eat it with your salads. Olives are great for salads and also a delicious and healthy snack. You may also make olive tapenade, a tasty olive spread that goes well with a wide variety of foods. Lastly, pesto is one of my absolute favorites. You can make this on your own quite easily, or you can buy it premade in a jar.

Proteins: All of the proteins you eat will come from vegetables. You should eat a variety of legumes such as chickpeas, beans, and lentils. Buy them dry and soak and boil them yourself rather than buying the prepackaged and processed kind.

• Quinoa is a good source of protein and makes a great ingredient in salads. Brown rice is also okay in small quantities. There are also several kinds of pasta and noodles that are made out of rice. For breakfast, you can make muesli or breakfast porridge out of buckwheat. You will also be consuming a small amount of protein when you eat nuts and seeds.

• Algae is a great source of protein, and it makes an excellent addition to salads. You buy it dry and soak it before you add it to your meal.

• The only animal-derived protein you will be eating will come from goat's milk and sheep's milk cheeses. You may choose freely between feta cheese, halluomi, chèvre, pecorino, manchego, and cream cheese.

Carbohydrates: You may eat as many vegetables, lettuces, root vegetables, fruits, and berries as you like. Always choose organic when possible. Frozen or dried vegetables and fruits are also perfectly fine so long as you avoid preservatives. Eat good quantities of members of the kale family, such as broccoli, cauliflower, red or white kale, and Brussels sprouts, as they are particularly rich in antioxidants.

For added taste: Drop prepackaged spice blends, ketchup, and sweet chili sauce. Instead you should use vinegar, Dijon mustard, tomato paste, pesto, soy sauce, ajvar, sundried tomatoes, capers, lemon, lime, ginger, garlic, spices, dried and fresh herbs, and bouillon without trans fats.

EAT RARELY

• Potatoes • Butter • Eggs

AVOID

• Processed and refined foods • Hydrogenated vegetable oils • Alcohol • Coffee • Black tea • Sugar and sweeteners • Red meat • White meat • Fish • Seafood • Wheat • Oats • Rye • Spelt/Dinkel • Grains • Painkillers

TWO-WEEK DETOX MENU

Day 1
Asian quinoa salad with coconut, p. 77
Raw power soup, p. 101

Day 2
Cauliflower tabouleh with halloumi and mint guacamole, p. 64
Ajvar and feta cheese pizza, p. 79

Day 3
Eggplant slices with chèvre chaud, p. 95
Quinoa salad with halloumi and pomegranate, p. 55

Day 4
Rice salad, p. 63
Roasted bell pepper soup with cress and goji berries, p. 106

Day 5
Rice noodles with coconut milk, p. 86
Roasted root vegetables with feta cheese, p. 89

Day 6
Root vegetable soup with saffron, p. 105
Beet quinoa with pea pesto, p. 52

Day 7
Falafel lettuce wraps, p. 84
Buckwheat rotini with warm tomato sauce, p. 83

Day 8
Tomato soup with pesto-marinated feta cheese, p. 98
Sprout salad with yellow beets and goat cheese, p. 71

Day 9
Summer salad with citrus dressing, p. 60
Mini eggplant, squash, and goat cheese towers with pine nut crust, p. 92

Day 10
Bean salad with arugula crème. p. 59
Chantarelle soup with rice noodles, p. 102

Day 11
Sweet potato soup with halloumi skewers, p. 105
Saffron quinoa with raisins and pomegranate, p. 67

Day 12
Fruity quinoa salad with mint pesto, p. 56
Stuffed rice leaves, p. 90

Day 13
Squash tagliatelle with feta cheese, nuts, and pesto, p. 51
Sweet potato pie with guacamole and tomatoes, p. 73

Day 14
Marinated beets with feta cheese, p. 77
Spinach and broccoli soup with pecorino cheese, p. 98

Breakfasts:
½ cup (1 dl) soy yogurt with ¼ cup (½ dl) detox
muesli, p. 20
Detox smoothie and fruit
plate, pp. 43, 24
Seed roll sandwich with bell peppers and pecorino cheese, p. 29
Raw porridge with fruit and
nuts, p. 24
Buckwheat porridge with cinnamon and cardamom, p. 23

Snacks:
Everything drink, p. 43
Avocado tart, p. 60
Seed and fig bar, p. 31
Seed crisp bread, p. 31
Miso soup, p. 101
Baked goat cheese with nuts and dried fruit, p. 32

Something Sweet:
Avocado and chocolate
mousse, p. 110
Banana mousse with chocolate and roasted coconut, p. 118
Fudge with passion fruit, p. 113
Almond muffins with blueberries and mango, p. 114
Health buns, p. 35

BREAKFAST

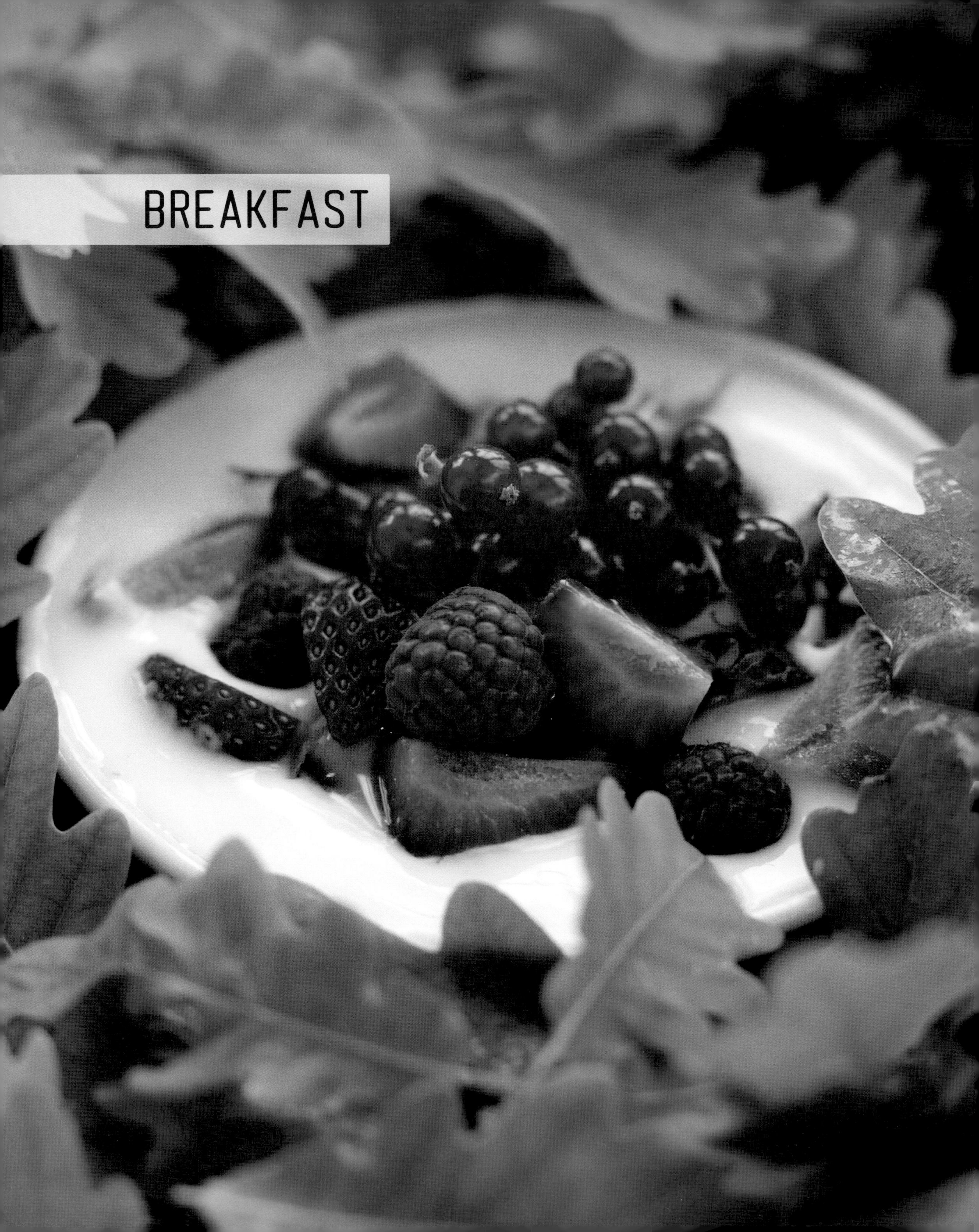

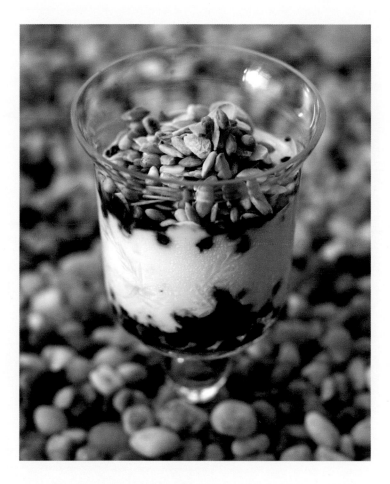

Soy yogurt with red berries

<u>1 serving</u>
¾ cup (1 ½ dl) plain soy yogurt
½ cup (1 dl) strawberries, sliced
¼ cup (½ dl) raspberries

Pour the yogurt in a bowl and top with berries. Serve as is.

Soy yogurt with blueberries and seeds

<u>1 serving</u>
¾ cup (1 ½ dl) plain soy yogurt
½ cup (1 dl) blueberries
¼ cup (½ dl) roasted mixed seeds and nuts, such as sunflower seeds, flaxseeds, pine nuts, almonds, and pumpkin seeds

Pour the yogurt in a bowl. Top with the berries, nuts, and seeds. Serve as is.

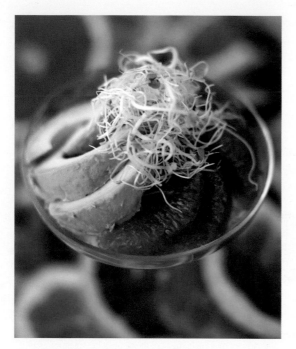

Avocado and grapefruit breakfast

<u>1 serving</u>
A luxurious breakfast packed with healthy fats and antioxidants.

1 avocado
1 grapefruit
½ cup (1 dl) alfalfa sprouts

Peel and slice the avocado. Peel the grapefruit and remove the flesh from the skin walls using a sharp knife. Place the avocado and grapefruit in a glass and top with the alfalfa sprouts.

Detox muesli

<u>1 batch</u>
A delicious, gluten-free muesli packed with nutrients. Serve with plain soy yogurt.

9 oz (250 g) whole buckwheat
½ cup (1 dl) sunflower seeds
9 oz (250 g) crushed buckwheat
1 ⅓ cups (100 g) flaked coconut
1 cup (150 g) chopped almonds
1 cup (150 g) chopped hazelnuts
⅓ cup (¾ dl) flaxseeds
½ tbsp cinnamon
½ tbsp cardamom powder
½ tbsp vanilla powder
3 tbsp liquid honey
½ cup (1 dl) chopped dried apricots
½ cup (1 dl) chopped dried dates
½ cup (1 dl) dried goji berries
½ cup (1 dl) pumpkin seeds

Rinse the whole buckwheat in several changes of water then let it soak with the sunflower seeds overnight. Set the oven to 380 degrees (200 C). Drain the soaked buckwheat and sunflower seeds and stir together in a medium-sized bowl with the crushed buckwheat, coconut flakes, almonds, hazelnuts, flaxseeds, spices, and vanilla powder. Spread the mixture on a baking sheet, pour the honey on top, and mix. Roast the muesli on the middle rack of the oven for about 20 minutes. You may stir a couple of times to ensure that they are roasted evenly. After 20 minutes remove the sheet from the oven and add the dried fruit and pumpkin seeds. Store in a closed container.

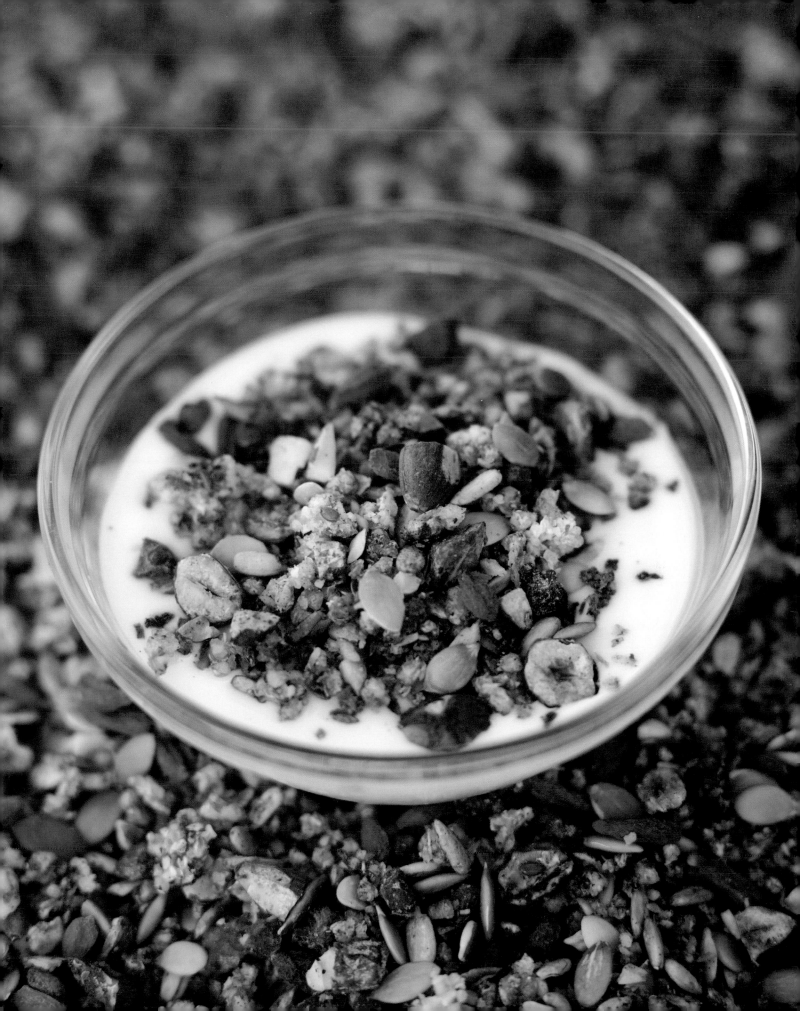

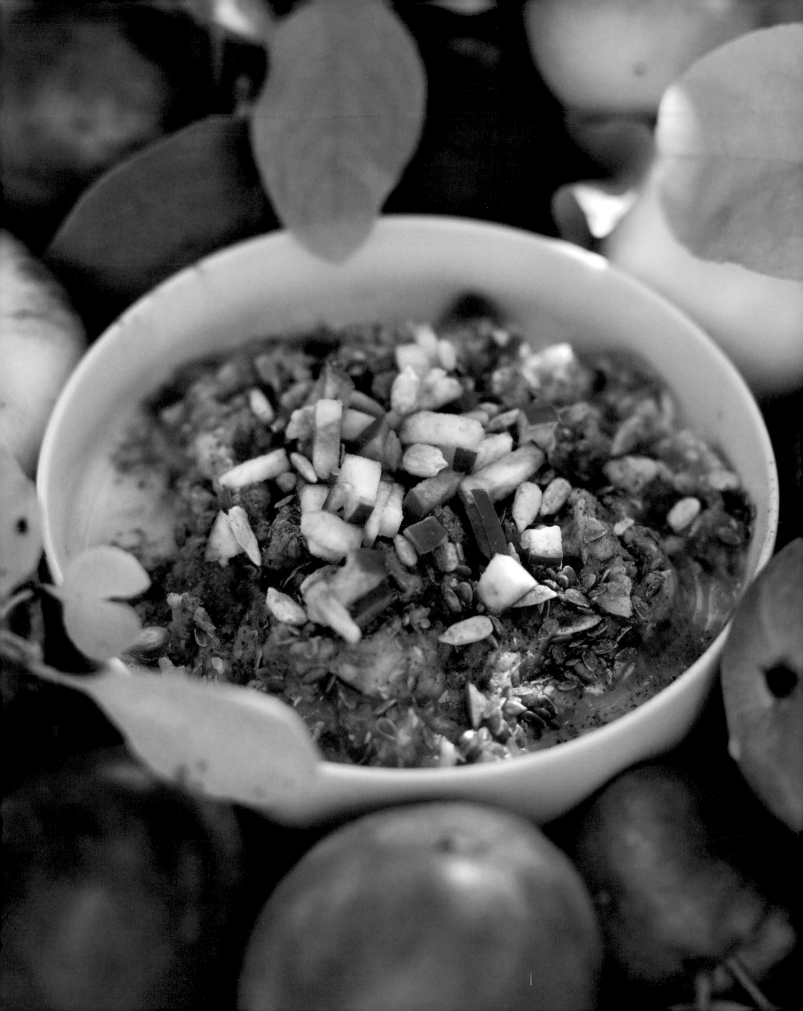

Buckwheat porridge with cinnamon and cardamom

<u>1 serving</u>

A delightful porridge that you can easily make multiple portions of in one session. Store in the fridge and add a little water and reheat every morning for breakfast.

½ cup (1 dl) buckwheat groats

3 dried apricots

½ apple

1 tsp flaxseeds

1 tbsp sunflower seeds

1 pinch of cinnamon

1 pinch of cardamom

1 cup (2 dl) water

1 pinch of salt

Serve with: grated apple, cinnamon, and soymilk

Boil the buckwheat in water and drain it before you place it back in the sauce pan. Roast it dry for a couple of minutes while you stir. Thinly slice the apricots and the apple. Simmer buckwheat with the apricots, apple, flaxseeds, sunflower seeds, cinnamon, cardamom, and the water over low heat. Add a pinch of salt and add more water if necessary. Cook for about 25 minutes. Top the porridge with grated apple and cinnamon. Serve with soymilk.

Cashew "cream cheese" with lemon and chives

<u>1 batch</u>

A rich cream similar to a cream cheese. Store in the fridge for up to one week.

1 cup (2 dl) cashew nuts

½ lemon

1 avocado

¼ cup (½ dl) chopped chives

Salt

Soak the nuts overnight. Drain and put them in a food processor. Grate the lemon peel and squeeze the juice from the lemon half in the processor as well. Peel and chop the avocado and add it with the chopped chives. Mix in the food processor until you have a creamy spread, adding water as needed. Add salt to taste.

Fruit plate

<u>1 serving</u>

A fresh fruit plate is an excellent way to start your day. If you want you may eat it with plain nuts.

½ mango
½ banana
1 slice of papaya
½ fig
½ passion fruit

Peel and chop the fruit and arrange on a plate.

Raw porridge with fruit and nuts

<u>1 serving</u>

You may make variations on this recipe by using other fruits, such as blueberries or mango.

1 small banana
1 ripe pear
¼ cup (½ dl) plain cashews
¼ cup (½ dl) hazelnuts
½ tbsp psyllium seeds*
½ tbsp sunflower seeds
1 tsp coconut oil

Serve with: coconut flakes, cinnamon, and soymilk

Peel the banana. Peel and chop the pear, removing the core. Place fruit, nuts, seeds, and coconut oil in a food processor and blend. Pour into a deep bowl and top with coconut flakes and cinnamon. Serve with soymilk.

*Psyllium seeds are available for purchase online and at health-food stores.

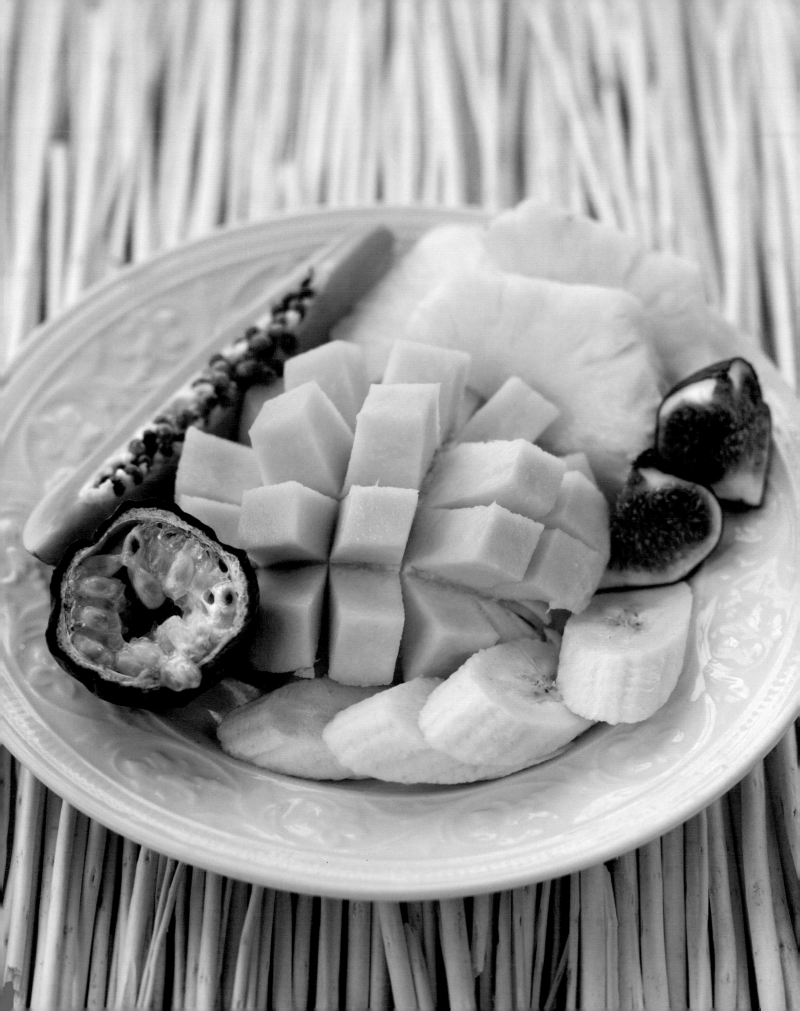

Almond and seed crackers

10 crackers

You can make good crackers free of bad carbohydrates by using seeds, nuts, and psyllium husks. Psyllium husks are good for colon cleansing and blood circulation, and they can be purchased online or at a health-food store. If you wish, you may add herbs or cinnamon and cardamom for flavor.

¼ cup (½ dl) flaxseeds
¼ cup (½ dl) almonds
1 tbsp sesame seeds
1 tbsp psyllium husks
2 eggs
2 tbsp coconut oil, extra virgin
½ tsp salt
Sesame seeds for garnish

Preheat the oven to 300 degrees (150 C). Mix the flaxseeds, almonds, and sesame seeds in a food processor. Pour the mixture in a mixing bowl and stir together with psyllium husks, beaten eggs, melted coconut oil, and salt. Roll out the dough and use a sharp knife to carve out circles, then transfer to a baking sheet. Sprinkle sesame seeds on top. Bake for 20 minutes. Turn the oven off, open the oven door, and let the crackers sit for an additional 30 minutes. Store the finished crackers in a cool place.

Seed rolls with carrots

8–10 rolls

It is possible to bake bread without the use of wheat flour. In this recipe, I've substituted flour with seeds. This bread may stored in the freezer. Eat it for breakfast or as an accompaniment to soup.

1 pound (½ kg) carrots
1 cup (2 dl) almonds
1 cup (2 dl) sunflower seeds, plus extra for topping
1 cup (2 dl) pumpkin seeds, plus extra for topping
½ cup (1 dl) flaxseeds
4 eggs

Set the oven to 340 degrees (175 C). Peel and grate the carrots. Mix the nuts and seeds with 1 ½ (3 dl) cups of the carrots. Add the rest of the carrots. Beat the eggs and mix with the rest of the ingredients. Divide the dough into pieces, shaping into small rolls, and place on a baking sheet. Sprinkle some pumpkin and sunflower seeds on top and bake for approximately 60 minutes.

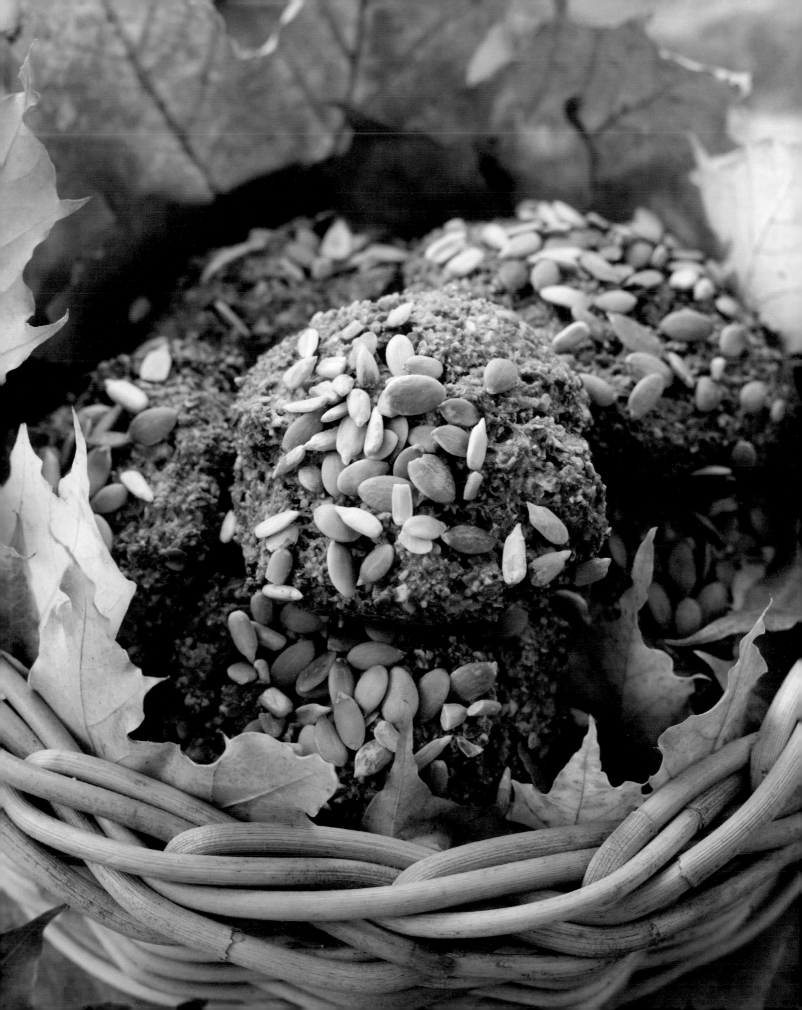

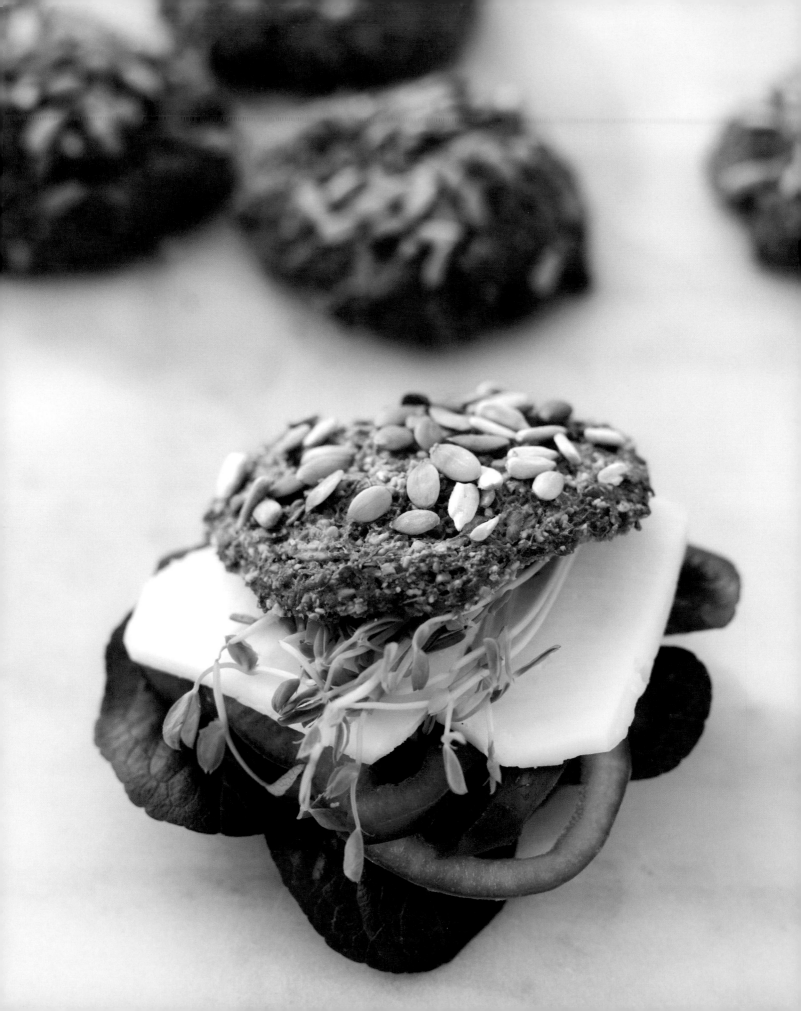

Seed roll sandwich with bell peppers and pecorino cheese

<u>1 serving</u>

1 seed roll, p. 26

1 lettuce leaf

2 slices bell peppers

2 slices pecorino cheese

Some pea shoots

Open the roll by slicing it horizontally. Place the lettuce, bell pepper, and cheese on the bottom half. Top with the pea shoots and close the sandwich with the other half to make a sandwich. Enjoy with a cup of tea.

Tomato crisp bread

<u>1 batch</u>

¼ cup (½ dl) sundried tomatoes

1 cup (2 dl) sunflower seeds

1 cup (2 dl) crushed flaxseeds

2 tomatoes

2 tbsp dried basil

1 pinch of sea salt

Soak the sundried tomatoes in ½ cup (1 dl) of water overnight. Soak the sunflower seeds overnight in a separate bowl. The next day, preheat a dehydrator to 100 degrees (40 C). Drain the sunflower seeds and put in a food processor. Add the sundried tomatoes and their water. Slice the fresh tomatoes, removing the core, then place in the food processor along with the flaxseeds, basil, and salt. Blend everything until it is evenly mixed. You should be able to shape it. Add more water if it is too hard, and if it's too thin add more flaxseeds. Spread the mixture on a medium baking sheet (or one of the trays included with your dehydrator) lined with parchment paper; spread it thin enough to cover the entire sheet. Bake in the dehydrator for 4–5 hours. Remove from the dehydrator and use a knife to carve into squares. Turn the squares upside down and return the sheet to the dehydrator. Bake it for an additional 4–5 hours. Let cool before serving. Store dry in a closed container.

SNACKS

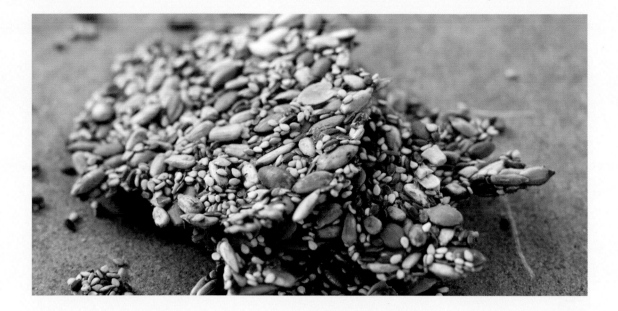

Seed and fig bar

About 20 bars

14 oz (400 g) sunflower seeds

7 oz (200 g) flaxseeds

7 oz (200 g) pumpkin seeds

5 oz (150 g) dried figs, chopped

7 oz (150 g) almonds

½ cup honey

1 tsp vanilla powder

4 eggs

Preheat the oven to 350 degrees (175 C). Mix the sunflower seeds, flaxseeds, pumpkin seeds, and chopped figs in a bowl. Grind the almonds into fine flour in a mixer. Add the almond meal, honey, and vanilla powder to the mix of seeds. Beat the eggs and pour into the bowl. Spread the mixture on a baking sheet lined with parchment paper. Bake on the bottom rack of the oven for approximately 20 minutes. Let cool and divide into portion pieces.

Seed crisp bread

1 batch

A tasty crisp bread that is well worth the time it takes to prepare it. The baked crisp bread will last for a couple of weeks, and it is both practical and luxurious to have a box of homemade crisp breads in your cupboard.

1 ½ cups (3 dl) flaxseeds

¼ cup (½ dl) sesame seeds

¼ cup (½ dl) sunflower seeds

¼ cup (½ dl) pumpkin seeds

1 ½ cups (3 dl) water

1 tsp vegetable broth

Mix the flaxseeds, sesame seeds, sunflower seeds, and pumpkin seeds with the water. Let sit for about 4 hours. Preheat a dehydrator to 104–113 degrees (40–45 C). Drain the seeds and place in a bowl with the broth. Mix together and spread a thin layer on a baking sheet (or one of the trays included with your dehydrator) lined with parchment paper. Let it bake in the dehydrator for about 8 hours. Break into smaller pieces and top with a spread such as cashew "cream cheese" (page 23).

31

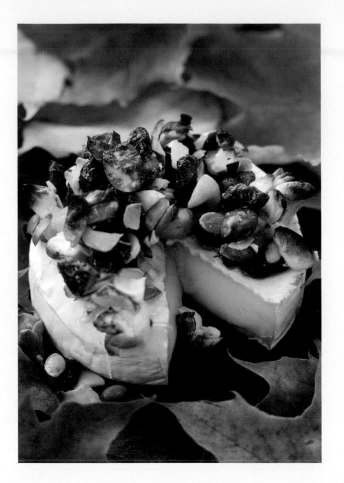

Baked goat cheese with nuts and dried fruit

<u>4 servings</u>

A piece of cheese with nuts and dried fruit for after dinner. Yummy!

1 slice goat brie cheese of any size
½ cup (1 dl) mixed nuts
1 tbsp cranberries
1 tbsp honey

Set the oven to 440 degrees (225 C). Place the cheese on a baking sheet lined with parchment paper and top with the nuts, cranberries, and honey. Bake for approximately 10 minutes.

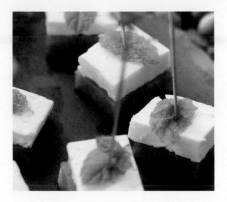

Feta and watermelon skewers

<u>2 servings</u>

Serve as a light meal or a refreshing snack.

¼ watermelon
2.5 oz (75 g) feta cheese
A few mint leaves

Carve the watermelon and feta into small, bite-sized squares. Stack one square of feta on each watermelon square, place a mint leaf on top, and stick on small skewers.

Endive leaf with goat cheese crème

<u>2 servings</u>

Serve as a luxurious snack.

1 endive
2 oz (50 g) feta cheese
1 fresh fig
1 tbsp dried cranberries
¼ cup (½ dl) roasted hazelnuts

Remove the hard ends of the stems of the endive and discard. Arrange the endive leaves on a serving platter. Top each leaf with some of the feta. Slice the fig and place on top of the cheese. Top with cranberries and hazelnuts.

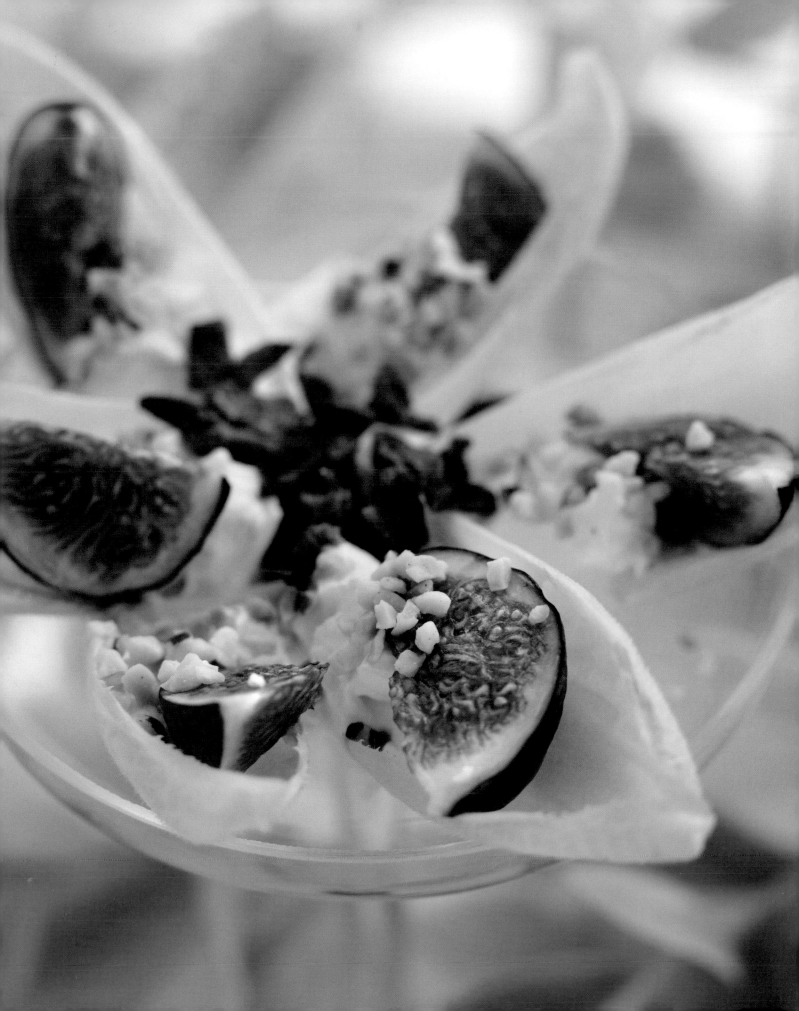

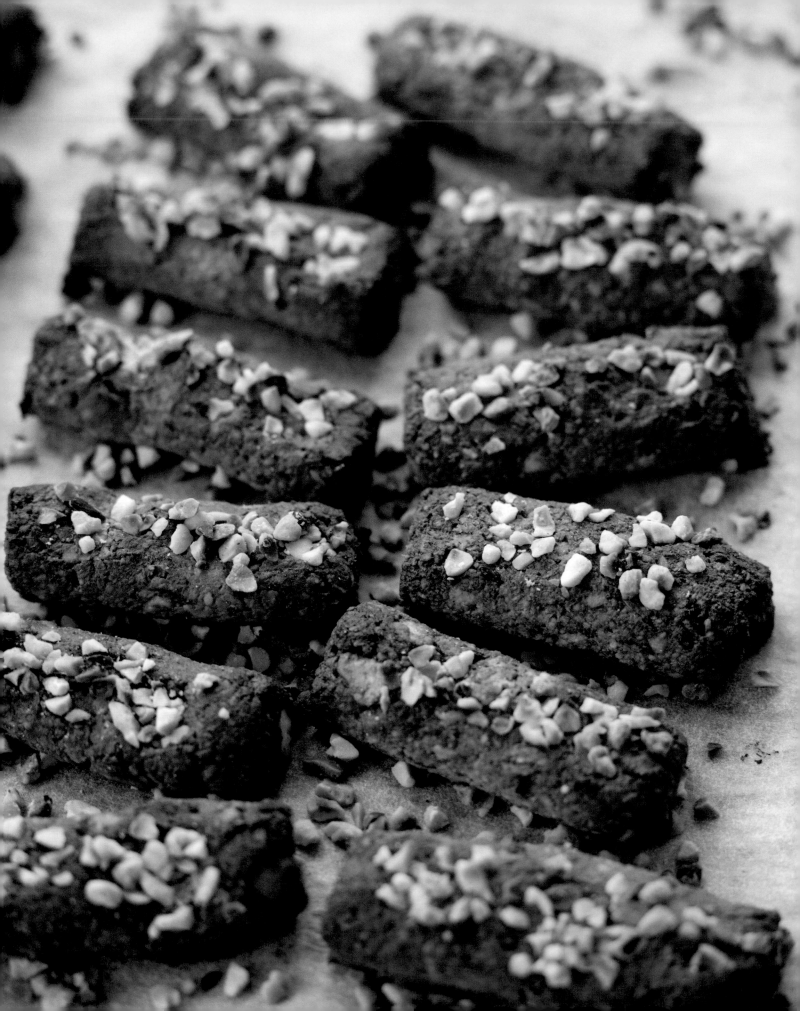

Mini nut biscuits

<u>20 biscuits</u>

7 oz (200 g) almonds

7 oz (200 g) hazelnuts, plus ¼ cup (½ dl) chopped hazelnuts for topping

10 dried dates

1 egg

Preheat the oven to 350 degrees (175 C). Grind the almonds and hazelnuts into fine flour. Chop the dates into smaller pieces, either by hand or using a mixer, and mix them with the flour and a beaten egg. Shape the dough into a long tube. Slice this into 2 ½-inch (7 cm) pieces and place the pieces on a baking sheet lined with parchment paper. Top with the chopped hazelnuts and bake for approximately 10 minutes.

Health buns

<u>25 buns</u>

Not only are these buns a sweet snack; they contain healthy fats, selenium, omega-3s, antioxidants, and vitamin C.

½ cup (1 dl) Brazil nuts

½ cup (1 dl) walnuts

¼ cup (½ dl) pumpkin seeds

¼ cup (½ dl) flaxseeds

1 cup (2 dl) soaked figs

1 banana

1 cup (2 dl) coconut flakes

Place the nuts, seeds, and figs in a food processor and blend into an even mixture. Add water if needed. Slice the banana into ½-inch (1-cm) pieces. Shape the nut mixture into buns and make a hole in each. Stuff a piece of banana into the holes and close up with the mixture. Dredge the buns in the coconut so that they are completely covered.

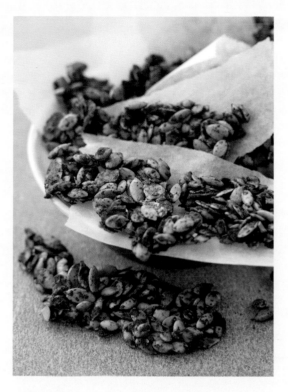

Pumpkin crisps with cinnamon

<u>1 batch</u>

Extremely tasty cookies that are rich in zinc and contain loads of omega-3s. The cookies may be served as a snack, a dessert, or as a topping for salads.

1 ½ cups (3 dl) pumpkin seeds

1 tbsp cinnamon

¼ cup (½ dl) honey

Soak the pumpkin seeds for 4 hours. Preheat a dehydrator to 113 degrees (45 C). Drain the seeds and mix with the cinnamon and honey in a bowl. Grease a small baking sheet (or one of the trays included with your dehydrator) with oil and spread the mixture on top. Bake for approximately 8 hours. Break into pieces and enjoy.

SMOOTHIES, JUICES & BEVERAGES

Currant and almond milk smoothie

<u>1 glass</u>
Almonds and currants comple-
ment each other wonderfully—
both creamy and sour.

½ cup (1 dl) almond milk
½ cup (1 dl) fresh or frozen
currants
2 ice cubes

Mix the ingredients in a blender.
Pour in a glass and drink immediately after making.

Cashew milk

<u>1 batch</u>
Make one batch at a time and
use in the preparation of different
smoothies.

5 dried apricots
2 ½ cups (5 dl) water
3.5 oz (100 g) plain cashews

Put the apricots in a blender
with the water. Let sit for about
5 minutes. Add the nuts and
blend into an even milk. Keeps for
about 5 days in the refrigerator.

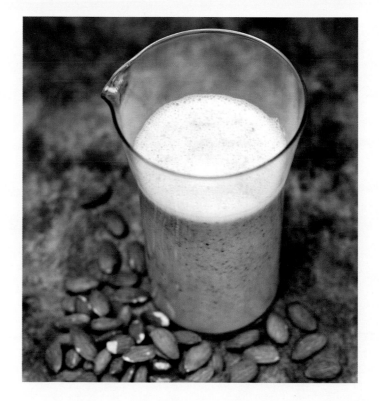

Almond milk

<u>1 batch</u>
Almond milk is good in smoothies or porridge.

4 dried figs
1 ½ cups (5 dl) water
13.5 oz (100 g) almonds

Put the figs in a blender with the water. Let it sit for 5 minutes. Add
the almonds and blend into an even milk. It will keep for 3–4 days
in the refrigerator.

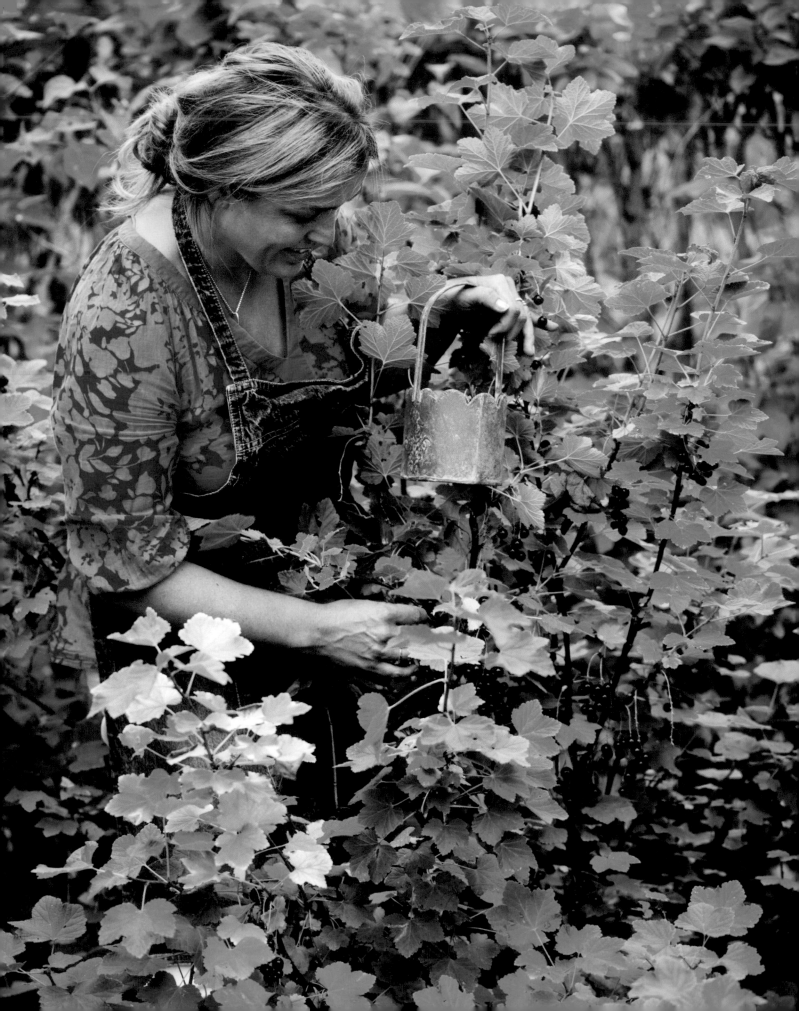

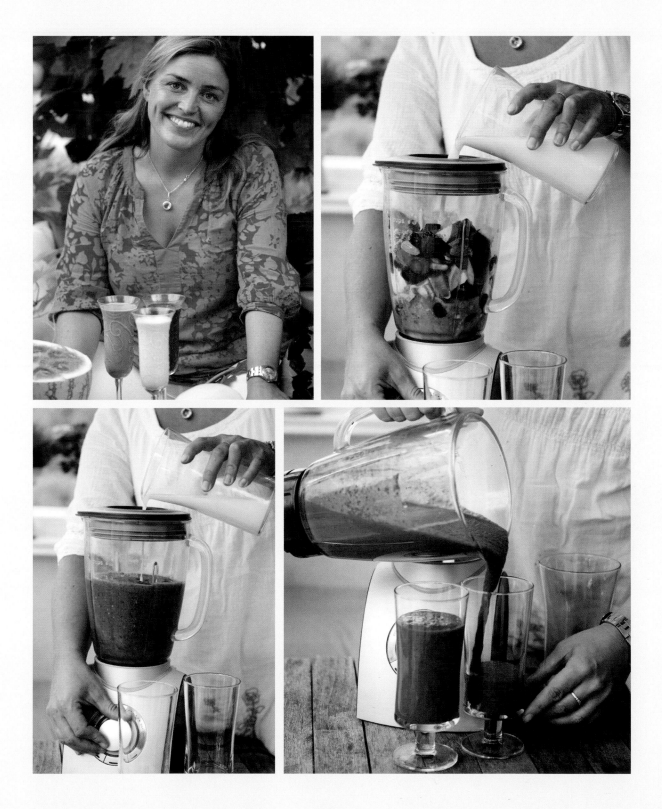

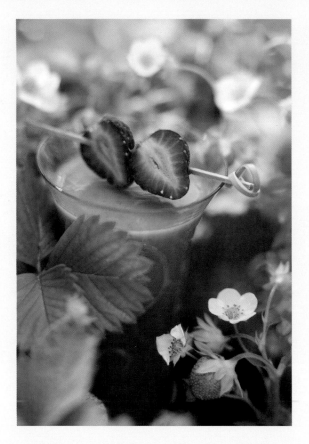

Cashew and blueberry smoothie

<u>1 serving</u>
½ cup (1 dl) cashew milk
½ cup (1 dl) frozen blueberries
½ cup (1 dl) watermelon, chopped
2 ice cubes

Mix all the ingredients using a blender. Pour in a glass and drink right away.

Cashew and cocoa smoothie

<u>1 serving</u>
¾ cup (1 ½ dl) cashew milk
1 tbsp cocoa
2 tbsp coconut flakes
2 ice cubes

Mix all the ingredients using a blender. Pour in a glass and drink right away.

Strawberry mango smoothie

<u>2 servings</u>
½ grapefruit
1 orange
½ banana
10 frozen strawberries
½ cup (1 dl) frozen chopped mango
2 ice cubes

Peel the grapefruit, orange, and banana. Place in a blender with the other ingredients and blend. Pour into two glasses and serve right away.

Cashew and mango smoothie

<u>1 serving</u>
½ cup (1 dl) cashew nut milk
½ cup (1 dl) frozen chopped mango
½ banana
2 ice cubes

Mix all of the ingredients using a blender. Pour in a glass and drink right away.

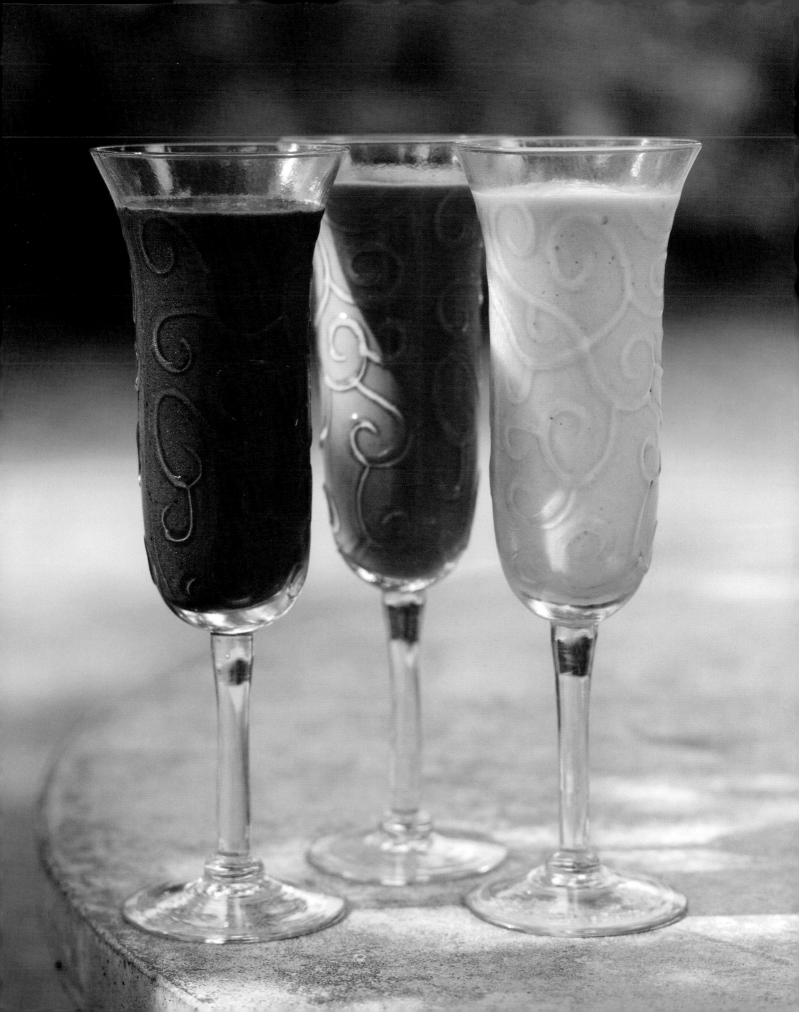

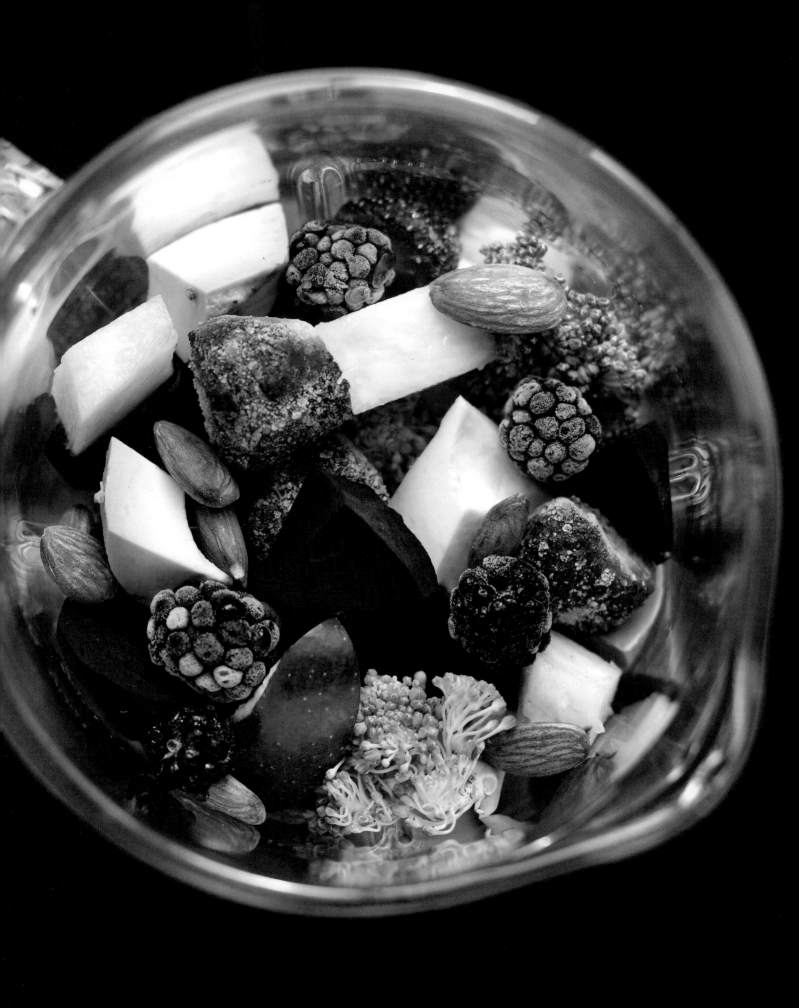

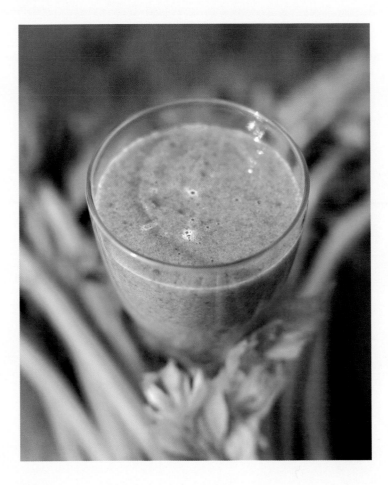

Everything drink

4 servings

1 avocado

2 beets

1 apple

1 cup (2 dl) pineapple, chopped

10 frozen strawberries

1.7 oz (50 g) almonds

5 florets broccoli

½ cup (1 dl) frozen blackberries

2 ice cubes

Cut open the avocado and remove the pit and skin. Peel the beets and chop into small pieces. Core and slice the apple. Mix all of the ingredients into a smoothie using a blender. Pour in four glasses and serve immediately.

Detox smoothie

2 servings

A delicious smoothie with a lot of iron and chlorophyll.

1 banana

2 stalks of celery

1 cup (2 dl) frozen spinach

½ cup (1 dl) orange juice

½ cup (1 dl) water

2 ice cubes

Peel the banana and chop the celery. Use a blender to mix the ingredients into a smoothie. Pour in two glasses and serve immediately.

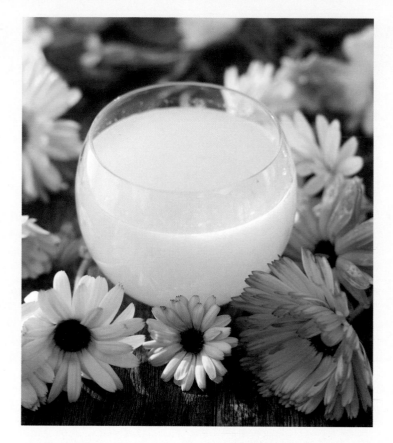

Pineapple and mango smoothie

2 servings
½ banana
1 orange
½ cup (1 dl) pineapple, chopped
½ cup (1 dl) papaya, chopped
Juice of ½ lime
2 ice cubes

Peel the banana and the orange and chop them into smaller pieces. Put them in a blender with the pineapple, papaya, and lime juice. Use a blender to mix into a smoothie. Add water if the mixture is too thick. Pour in two glasses and serve right away.

Raspberry temptation

2 servings
5 oz frozen raspberries
½ cup (1 dl) freshly squeezed grapefruit juice
2 tbsp agave syrup
2 ice cubes

Mix all the ingredients into a smoothie using a blender. Pour in two glasses and serve right away.

Lemonade

1 batch
Juice from 4 limes
Juice from 4 lemons
¼ cup (½ dl) agave syrup
5 ice cubes
5 cups sparkling water

Pour all of the ingredients into blender and mix for a few minutes. Pour in glasses and serve right away.

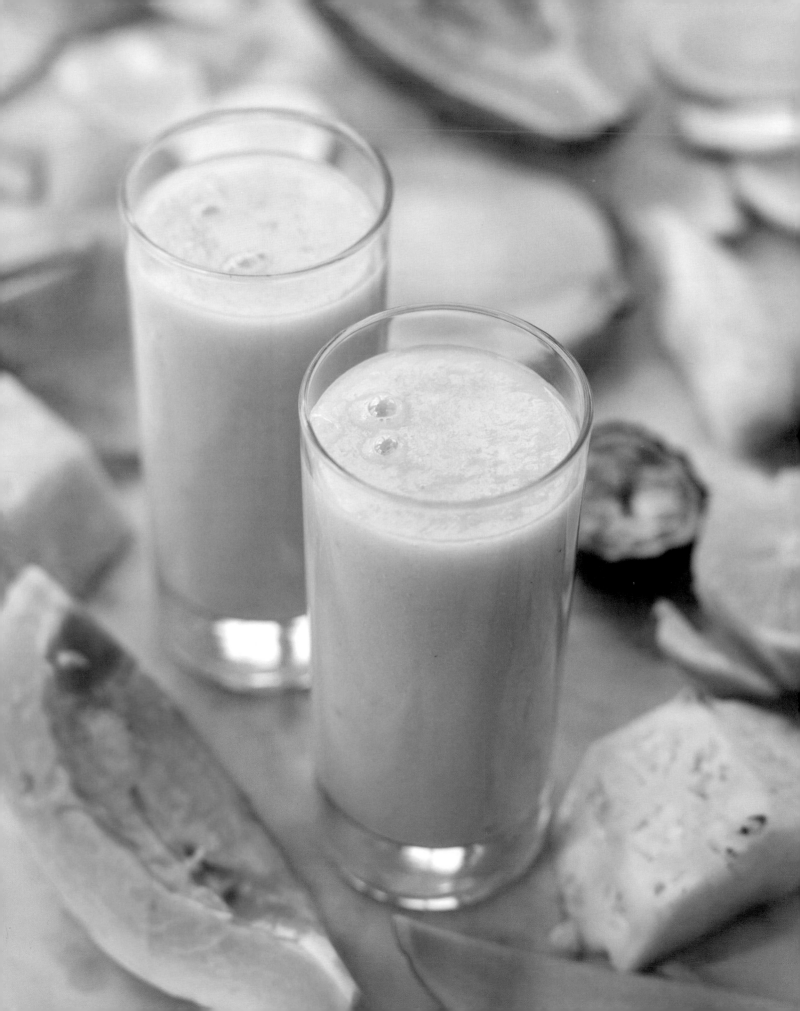

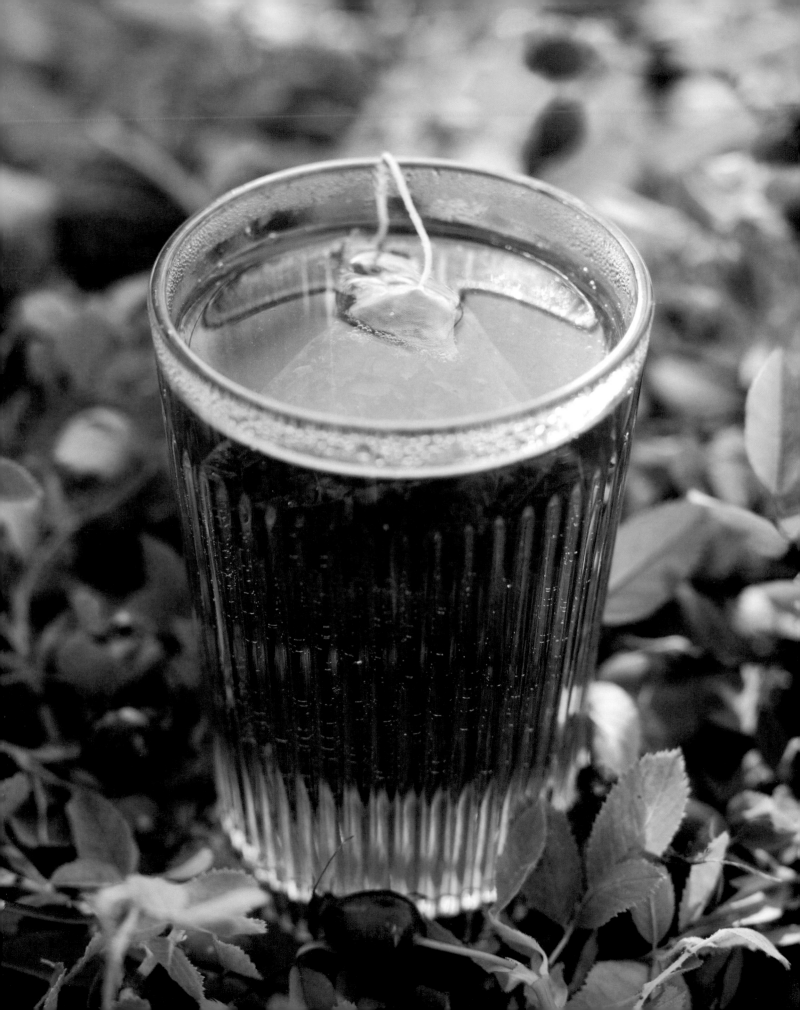

Dry rosehips to make your own rosehip tea.

Rosehips can be dried, ground, and used in soups, smoothies, and tea. Pick rosehips when they are ripe and rinse them carefully with water. Let them dry on a towel or sheet for a couple of days or until they are completely dry. You may also use a dehydrator to dry them at a low temperature (approximately 120 degrees F, 50 C) for 5–6 hours. Grind the rosehips and store in a cool, dry place.

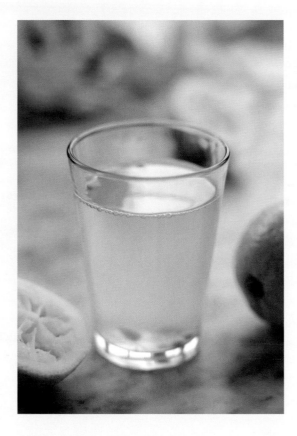

Rosehip tea

<u>1 cup</u>
1 tsp ground rosehips
1 cup (2 dl) boiling water
1 tsp honey

Water with lemon

<u>1 cup</u>
Start your day off with a glass of warm water and lemon to aid your kidneys in the cleansing process.

1 cup (2 dl) water
Juice of ¼ lemon

Heat the water in a pot and add the lemon juice. Let stand for a few minutes. Drink before breakfast.

Detox juices

Whenever you do a detox, it is crucial that you are able to make your own fruit and vegetable juices. The juices aid the body in the cleansing process while supplying it with nutrients such as vitamins, minerals, antioxidants, and fibers.

The easiest way to make vegetable juice is by using a juice press or a juice extractor. You can also use a blender, although this will most likely leave small bits of fruit in the liquid. I prefer to use a juice extractor. It can extract juice from almost any vegetable or fruit and it separates the pulp from the liquid.

Beet juice with berries

1 glass

3.5 oz (100 g) beets
3.5 oz (100 g) frozen blueberries
3.5 oz (100 g) frozen strawberries or raspberries
2 ice cubes

Juice the beets using a juicer (or blender) then pour the juice in a blender. Add the blueberries, strawberries, and/or raspberries and mix. Pour in a glass and garnish with strawberries. Drink right away.

Carrot-apple juice

1 serving

3 carrots
1 apple
⅓ inch (1 cm) fresh ginger
2 ice cubes

Juice all of the ingredients in a blender or juice extractor. Pour in a glass and drink right away.

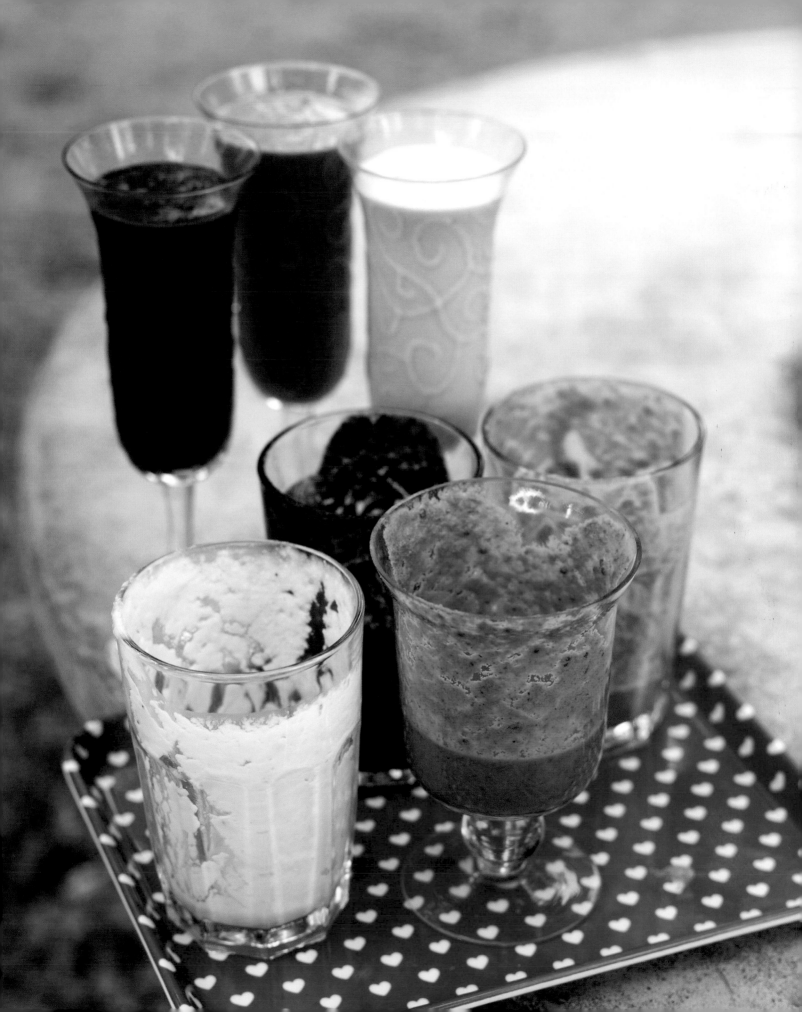

COLD DISHES

Squash tagliatelle with feta cheese, nuts, and pesto

<u>4 servings</u>
1–2 yellow summer squash, zucchini, or a combination of the two
2 carrots
5 oz (150 g) feta cheese
¼ cup (½ dl) walnuts
¼ cup (½ dl) cranberries

Basil and dill pesto
<u>1 batch</u>
1 bunch basil
5 sprigs of dill
1 garlic clove
Juice of ½ lemon
1.7 oz (50 g) pecorino cheese
½ cup (1 dl) olive oil
Salt and black pepper
Physalis and sliced lemon for garnish

Start off by making the pesto. Mix all of the ingredients except the olive oil in a food processor. Slowly pour the oil into the mixture and keep blending until it reaches an even consistency. Add salt and pepper according to taste. Store in the refrigerator.

Peel the squash and carrots into "tagliatelle" with the help of a potato peeler. Place on a plate. Pour the pesto over the tagliatelle and toss it lightly so that the pesto is evenly distributed. Sprinkle walnuts, cranberries, and crumbles of feta cheese on top. Garnish with physalis and sliced lemon.

Beet quinoa with pea pesto

<u>4 servings</u>

Furikake is a Japanese condiment that consists of black and white sesame seeds and edible algae. It's salt-free, making it a perfect way to add flavor to almost any dish!

4 small beets
1 ½ cups (3 dl) quinoa
2 tbsp olive oil
Juice of 1 lemon
Salt and black pepper
5 oz (150 g) peapods
1 cup (2 dl) frozen peas
2.5 oz (70 g) arugula
Furikake for topping

Pea pesto

<u>1 batch</u>
3.5 oz (100 g) almonds
1 cup (2 dl) frozen peas
Juice of 1 lemon
1 garlic clove
1 cup (2 dl) canola oil
Salt and black pepper

Begin by making the pea pesto. Mix the almonds, peas, lemon juice, and garlic in a food processor. Slowly pour the oil into the mixture and keep blending until it achieves an even consistency. Add salt and pepper to taste.

Boil the beets in lightly salted water for approximately 40 minutes. Drain the beets, then peel and chop them. Rinse the quinoa and boil it in lightly salted water for approximately 13 minutes. Drain the quinoa and mix with the beets. Drizzle the olive oil and lemon juice on top, then add salt and pepper. Slice the peapods and mix with the salad and the peas. Rinse the arugula and arrange it on a plate, top with the beet quinoa salad, and serve with the pea pesto. Top the dish with furikake.

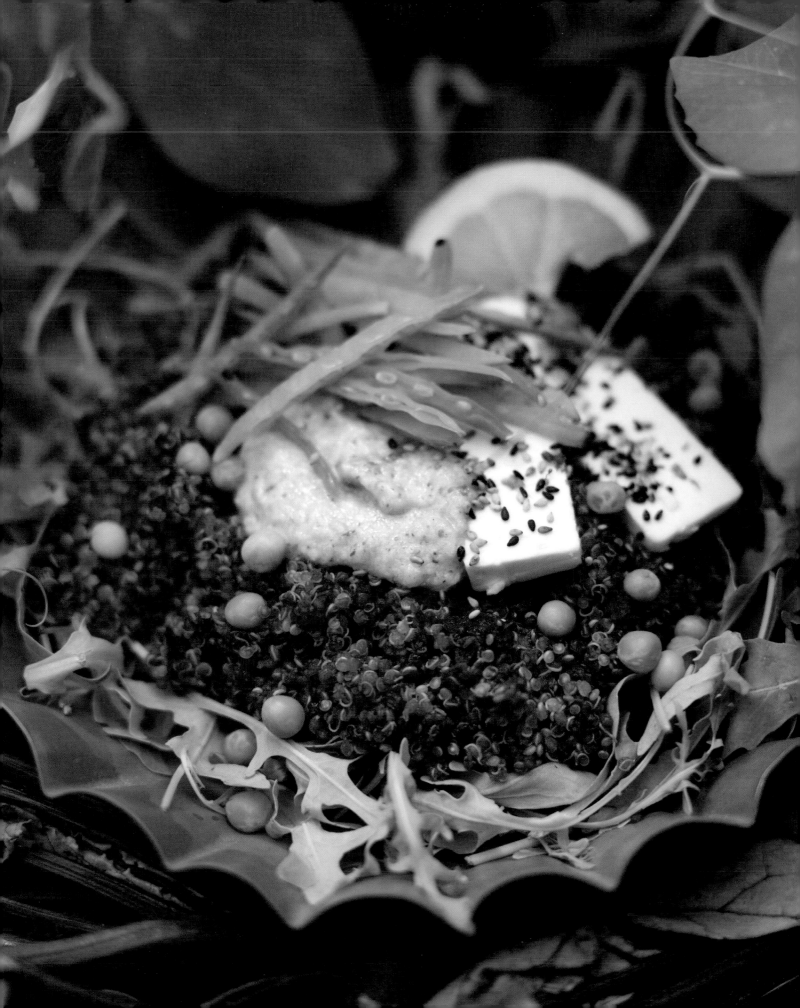

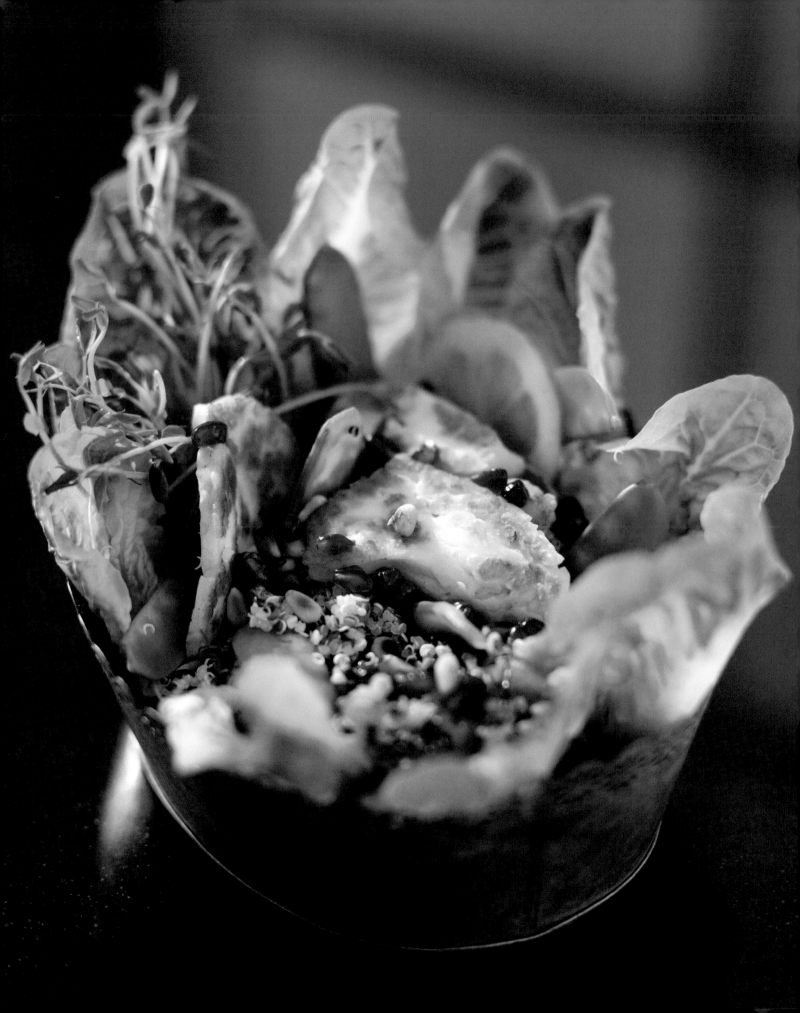

Quinoa salad with halloumi and pomegranate

<u>4 servings</u>

½ cup (1 dl) red quinoa

½ cup (1 dl) black quinoa

½ cup (1 dl) white quinoa

¼ cup (½ dl) mixed herbs (dill, basil, chives, etc.)

1 cup (2 dl) frozen peas

Salt and black pepper

2 tbsp olive oil

1 lemon

1 head of lettuce

2.5 oz (75 g) peapods

2.5 oz (75 g) pea shoots

½ pomegranate

5 oz (150 g) halloumi cheese

1 tbsp olive oil

5 oz (150 g) pine nuts for topping

Rinse the quinoa and boil for 13 minutes. You may boil the red and black quinoa together, but the white needs to be boiled in a separate pot. Drain and place in a large bowl. Add herbs and peas and season with salt and pepper. Drizzle the olive oil and lemon juice over the salad. Top with lettuce, peapods, and pea shoots. Garnish with pomegranate. Slice the halloumi about half an inch wide and fry the slices in oil. Add these to the salad. Heat a dry cooking pan and roast the pine nuts until they are lightly toasted. Sprinkle the pine nuts over the salad and serve.

Fruity quinoa salad with mint pesto

<u>4 servings</u>
1 ½ cups (3 dl) quinoa
2 red grapefruit
2 avocado
1 Pakistani mango
1 tbsp olive oil
½ lemon
Salt and pepper

Mint pesto
<u>1 batch</u>
1 bunch mint leaves
¼ cup (½ dl) pine nuts
Juice of 1 lime
½ cup (1 dl) olive oil
Salt and black pepper

Topping: ¼ cup (½ dl) roasted pine nuts, sunflower seeds, and mint leaves

Begin by making the mint pesto. Mix the mint leaves, pine nuts, and lime juice in a food processor. Slowly add the oil to the mixture and continue blending until it achieves an even consistency. Add salt and pepper to taste.

Rinse the quinoa and boil in lightly salted water for 13 minutes. Supreme the grapefruit and peel and slice the avocado and mango. Drain the quinoa and mix in the grapefruit, avocado, and mango. Drizzle the salad with the olive oil and lemon juice, then add salt and pepper. Heat a dry cooking pan and roast the pine nuts until they are light brown. Finally, sprinkle the pine nuts, sunflower seeds, and mint on top and serve with the mint pesto.

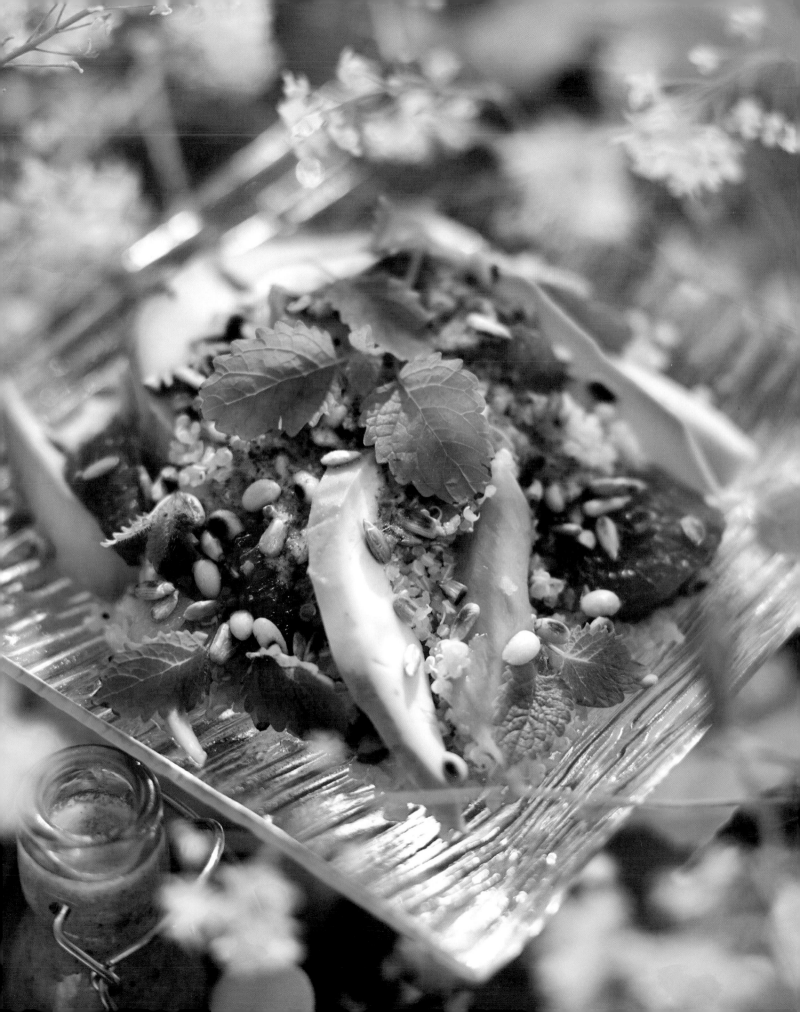

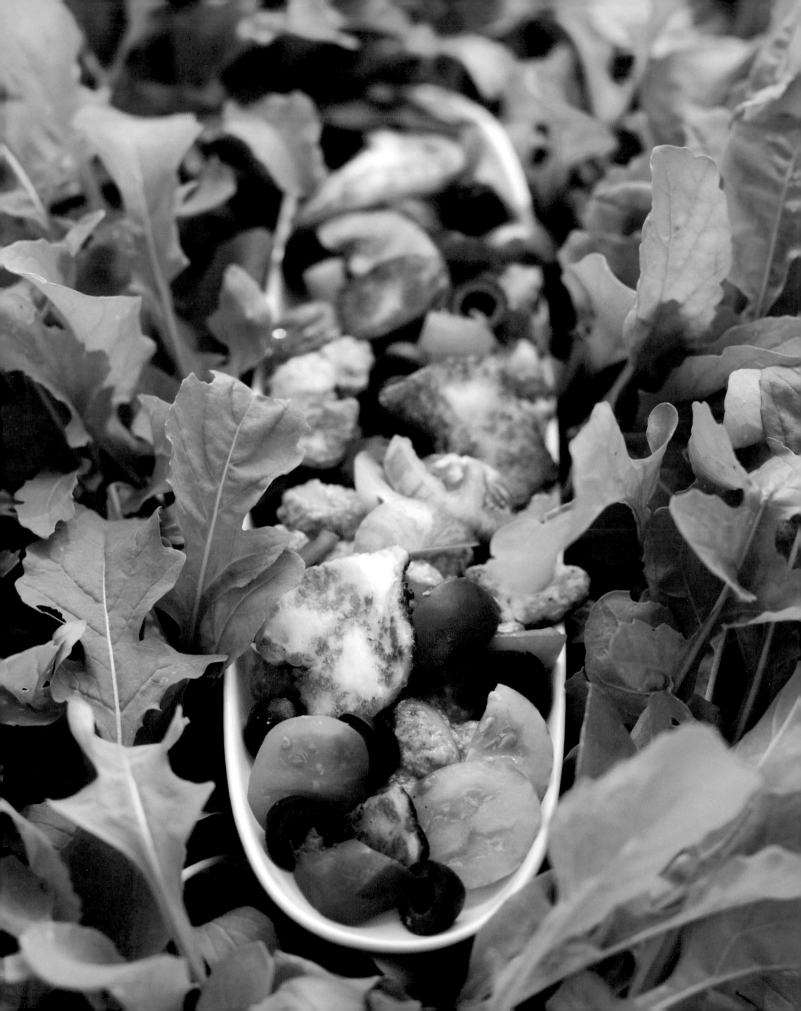

Bean salad with arugula crème

<u>4 servings</u>
2 cans white beans
½ red onion
8–9 oz (250 g) tomatoes of various colors
8–9 oz (250 g) halloumi cheese
1 tbsp olive oil
2.5 oz (70 g) arugula
3.5 oz (100 g) canned, pitted black olives
Salt and black pepper

Arugula crème
<u>1 batch</u>
3.5 oz (100 g) arugula
½ cup (1 dl) walnuts
½ cup (1 dl) cashews
1 garlic clove
½ red onion
¼ cup (½ dl) olive oil
½ cup (1 dl) canola oil
1 tsp honey
Salt and black pepper

Begin by making the arugula crème. Mix arugula, walnuts, cashews, and peeled and chopped onion and garlic in a food processor. Slowly pour the olive oil, canola oil, and honey into the mixture and blend it all together. Season with salt and pepper.

Rinse and drain the beans, then mix with the arugula crème. Peel and finely chop the red onion. Dice the tomatoes. Slice the cheese and fry it in oil for a few minutes on each side. Place the bean salad on a plate. Scatter the arugula about the dish. Top with the tomatoes, olives, and halloumi cheese, and season with salt and pepper.

Summer salad with citrus dressing

4 servings
2.5 oz (75 g) shelled hazelnuts

5 oz (150 g) mixed lettuce

1 red onion

2 avocados

1 lemon

Salt

8–9 oz (250 g) strawberries

10 oz (300 g) feta cheese

Fresh dill

2 tbsp olive oil

1 tbsp balsamic vinegar

Roast the hazelnuts in a dry frying pan. Rinse the lettuce and arrange it on a plate. Peel and slice the onion and avocados. Place the onion and the hazelnuts on top of the lettuce and squeeze the juice from half of the lemon over the avocado. Season with salt. Rinse and slice the strawberries and add them to the salad. Top it off with crumbled feta cheese. Slice the other half of the lemon and use as a garnish along with the dill. Drizzle the salad with olive oil and balsamic vinegar and serve right away.

Avocado tart

4 servings

2 large avocados

½ lemon

1.7 oz (50 g) goat cheese

½ small zucchini

1 tbsp olive oil

Salt and pepper

5 radishes

Spinach leaves

2 tbsp shelled hemp seeds

Cut open each avocado and remove the pits. Drizzle the lemon juice over the avocados. Fill the halves with goat cheese. Cut the squash in two and chop it into smaller pieces. Sauté in oil over low heat for a few minutes in a frying pan, stirring occasionally. Add salt and pepper. Rinse and slice the radishes. Add the squash and radishes to the avocado halves and top it off with the spinach leaves and hemp seeds.

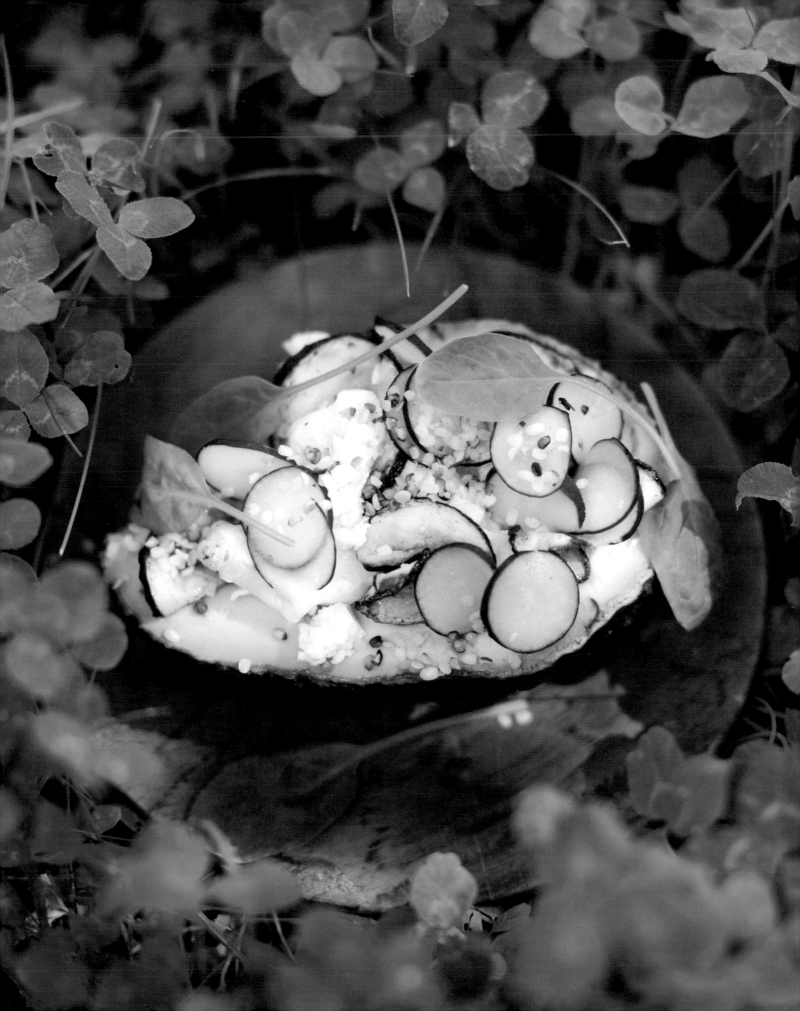

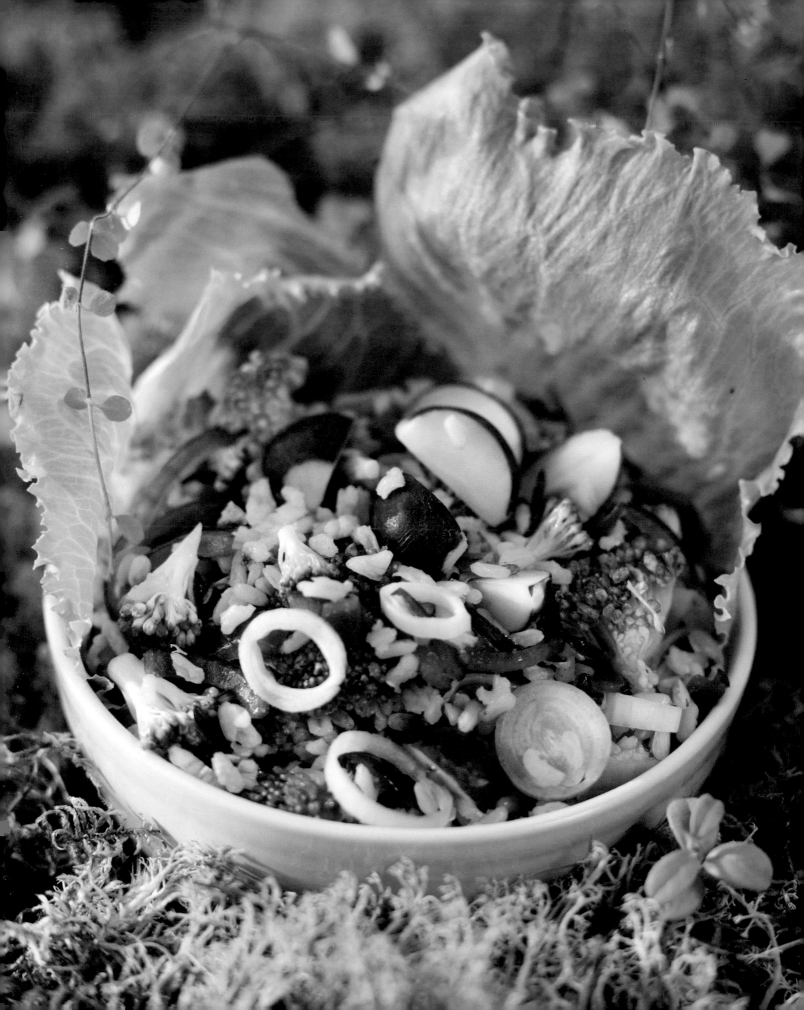

Rice salad

4 servings
1 ½ cups (3 dl) brown rice

½ cup (1 dl) wild rice

1 red onion

½ head of broccoli

1 tbsp olive oil

2 tbsp chopped fresh parsley

Juice of ½ lemon

Salt and black pepper

2 inches (5 cm) leek

1 can roasted bell peppers

½ handful radishes

Lettuce

Boil the rice in lightly salted water for about 30 minutes or until it is properly cooked. Peel and slice the red onion. Carve the broccoli into small florets. Fry the broccoli and onion for a few minutes in oil. Add the drained rice, the parsley, and lemon juice. Season with salt and pepper. Slice the leek and chop the bell peppers into small pieces. Mix with the rice salad and add sliced radishes. Serve with a lettuce leaf and perhaps some olive tapenade, p. 121.

Cauliflower tabbouleh with halloumi and mint guacamole

4 servings
1 cauliflower
Juice of 1 lemon
1 tbsp olive oil
½ cup (1 dl) chopped parsley
¼ cup (½ dl) chopped mint leaves
Salt and black pepper
About 8–9 oz (250 g) cherry tomatoes
5 oz (150 g) halloumi cheese
1 tbsp olive oil

Mint guacamole

1 batch
2 ripe avocados
½–1 pressed garlic clove
1 bunch of mint leaves
1 tbsp lemon juice
Salt and black pepper

Sliced lemon and mint leaves for garnish

Begin by making the mint guacamole. Peel and slice the avocados. Mix the avocado, garlic, and mint leaves into an even spread. Add lemon juice, salt, and pepper.

Break the cauliflower into small florets and place in a food processor. Mix until they achieve a grainy consistency, like thick mashed potatoes. Place in a bowl and add the lemon juice, olive oil, parsley, and mint leaves and stir until they are evenly distributed. Season with salt and pepper. Slice the tomatoes and the halloumi cheese. Use a frying pan to fry the cheese lightly on both sides. Serve the cauliflower tabbouleh with the cherry tomatoes, halloumi, sliced lemon, mint leaves, and mint guacamole.

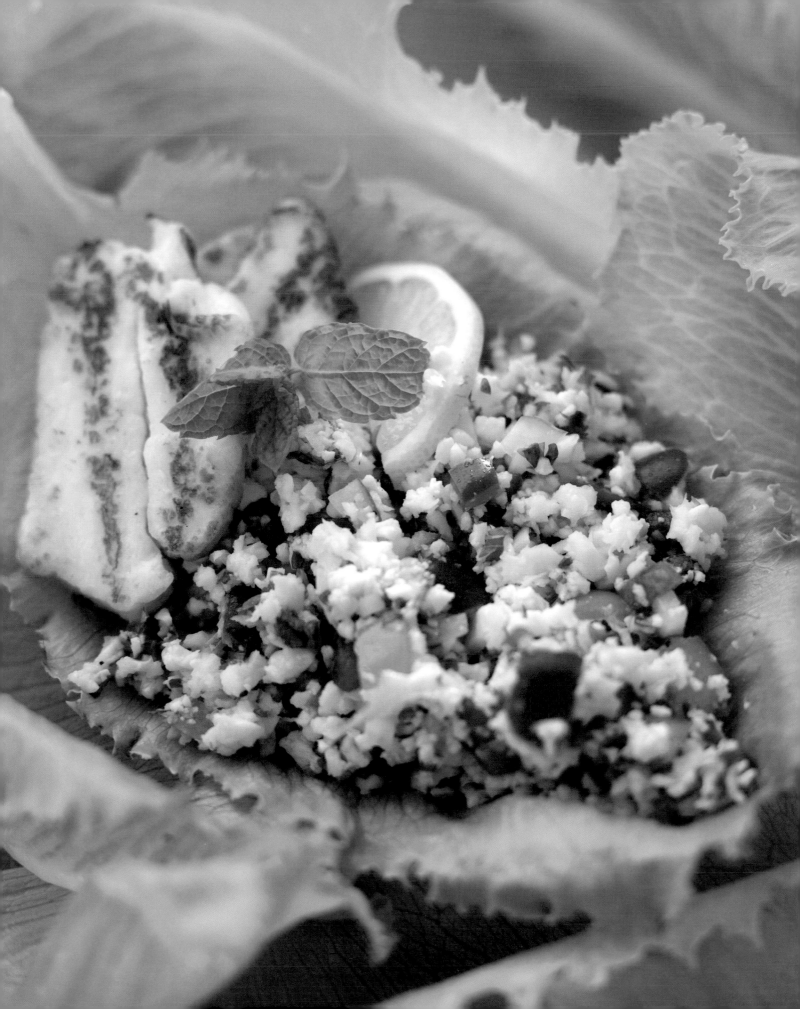

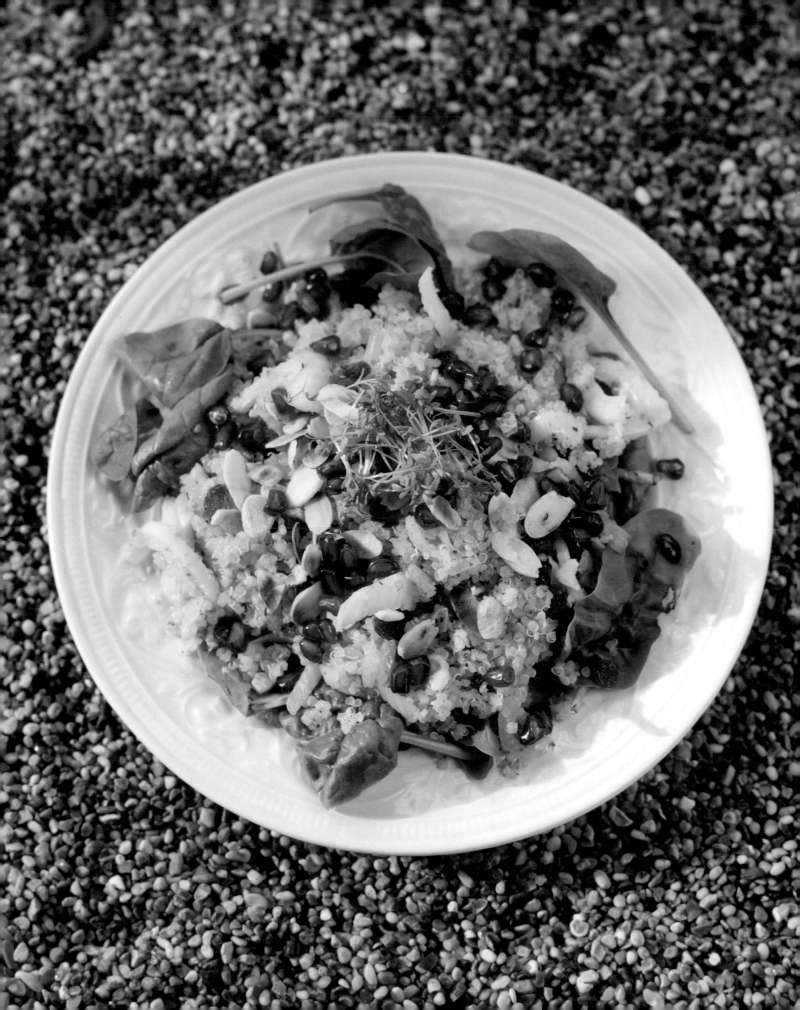

Saffron quinoa with raisins and pomegranate

4 servings

This salad may be served warm, lukewarm, or cold—it will be just as good.

1 yellow onion

1 fennel bulb

¼ tsp saffron

1 ½ cups (3 dl) white quinoa

1 tbsp vegetable bouillon

3 cups (6 dl) water

½ cup (1 dl) raisins

¼ cup chopped parsley

2.5 oz (70 g) fresh spinach leaves

Salt and black pepper

¼ cup (½ dl) shelled almonds, some pomegranate kernels, and a little watercress for garnish

Peel and slice the onion and fennel. Heat some olive oil in a frying pan. Sauté the onion and fennel and add the saffron. Rinse the quinoa well and add to the pan. Stir for a few minutes. Pour the water and bouillon in the pan and let it boil for about 10 minutes. Keep stirring from time to time; the dish is finished when all of the liquid has cooked off. Add the raisins and parsley and season with salt and pepper. Place the spinach leaves on a large plate and pour the quinoa salad on top. Roast the almonds in a dry frying pan. Garnish the salad with the shelled almonds, pomegranate, and cress, and serve.

Algae salad with black lentils

<u>4 servings</u>
1 cup (2 dl) black lentils
1 oz (20 g) rice noodles
0.5 oz (15 g) dried, mixed algae
2 carrots
2 garlic cloves
1 tbsp grated fresh ginger
1 tbsp canola oil
1 tbsp sesame seeds
1 red chili
1 tbsp tamari soy sauce
3.5 oz (100 g) sugar snap peas
1 tbsp sesame oil
½ tbsp coriander
½ tbsp furikake
1 oz (30 g) Chinese cabbage

Boil the lentils in lightly salted water for about 20 minutes. Boil the noodles for about 5 minutes or follow the directions on the package. Soak the algae for 10 minutes. Peel the carrots then shave them into long, thin pieces using the peeler. Drain the lentils and noodles. Peel and grate the garlic and ginger. Mince the chili. Heat a frying pan and add canola oil. Add the garlic, ginger, sesame seeds, chili, tamari soy sauce, and rice noodles and sauté over medium heat for a few minutes. Remove the algae from the water and squeeze it so that the liquid is drained. Add the algae to the frying pan and let it sauté for a couple of minutes more. Add the sugar snaps and carrot strips. Pour the sesame oil over the vegetables and mix in the coriander and furikake. Serve with Chinese cabbage.

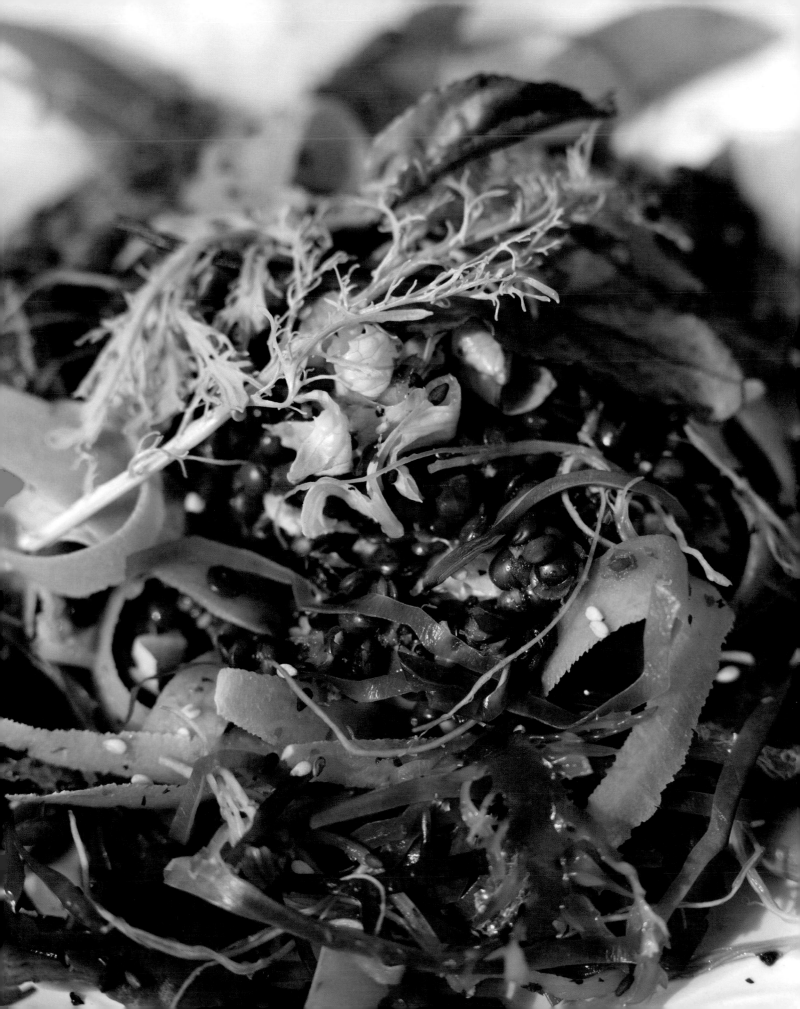

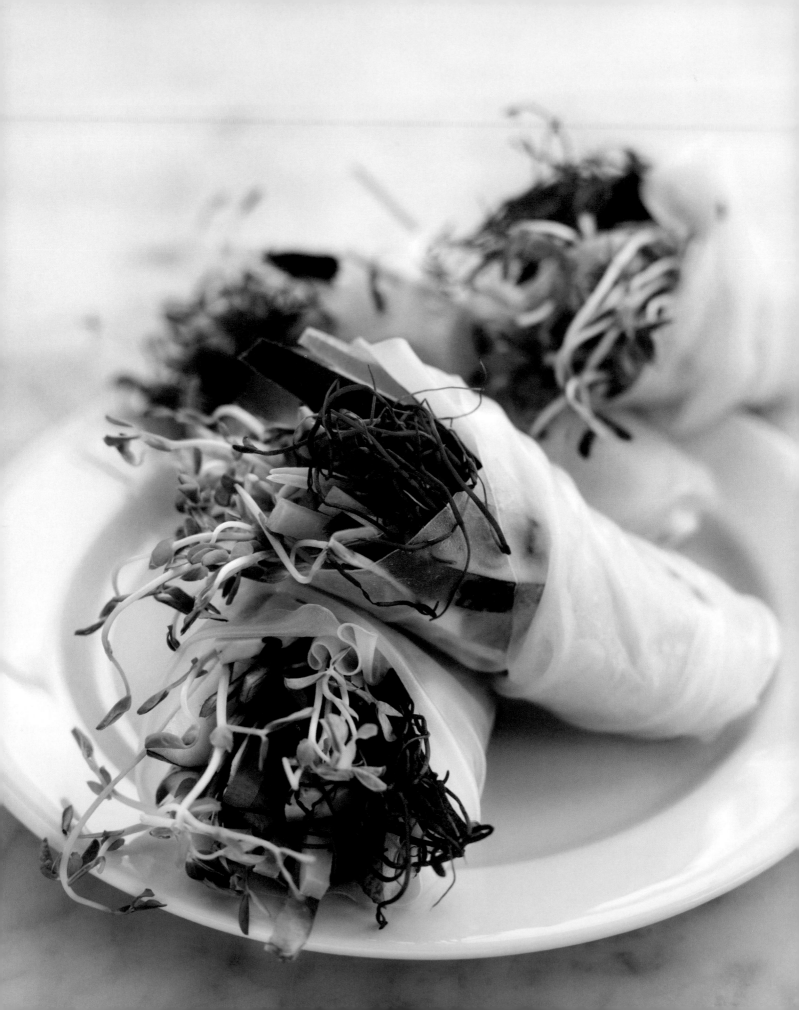

Rice leaves stuffed with fruits and vegetables

<u>4 servings</u>
1 avocado
1 carrot
1 peach
1 pear
3.5 oz (100 g) sugar snap peas
2 inches (5 cm) leek
8 rice leaves
½ cup (1 dl) mixed sprouts
(alfalfa sprouts and bean
sprouts)

Asian dipping sauce
<u>1 batch</u>
1–2 tbsp rice vinegar
1 tbsp light soy sauce
½ tsp sesame oil
2 tbsp canola oil
2 tbsp chopped coriander
½ tsp muscovado sugar
½ tsp sambal oelek (chili paste)
1 tbsp water

Mix all the ingredients for the dipping sauce together and refrigerate.

Cut the vegetables and fruits into long strips. Soak the rice leaves for about 30 seconds, until they become soft. Stuff them with the vegetables and fruit and fold the leaves to form a wrap. Top with the sprouts and serve with Asian dipping sauce.

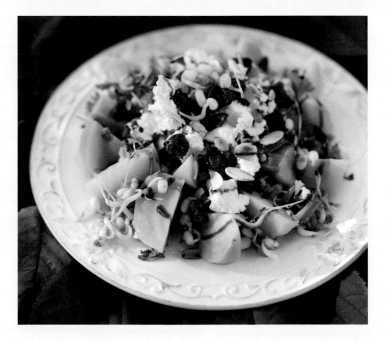

Sprout salad with yellow beets and goat cheese

<u>4 servings</u>
4 yellow beets
1 cup (2 dl) bean sprouts
¼ cup (½ dl) chopped parsley
2 tbsp olive oil
1 tbsp balsamic vinegar
5 oz (150 g) goat cheese
¼ cup (½ dl) dried cranberries
¼ cup (½ dl) mixed nuts and seeds (almond, sunflower seeds, pumpkin seeds, etc.)
Extra goat cheese, cranberries, nuts, and seeds for topping

Boil the yellow beets in lightly salted water for about 30 minutes or until they become soft. Cut into small wedges and place them in a bowl. Add the bean sprouts, parsley, olive oil, and vinegar and mix. Top with crumbled goat cheese, dried cranberries, nuts, and seeds.

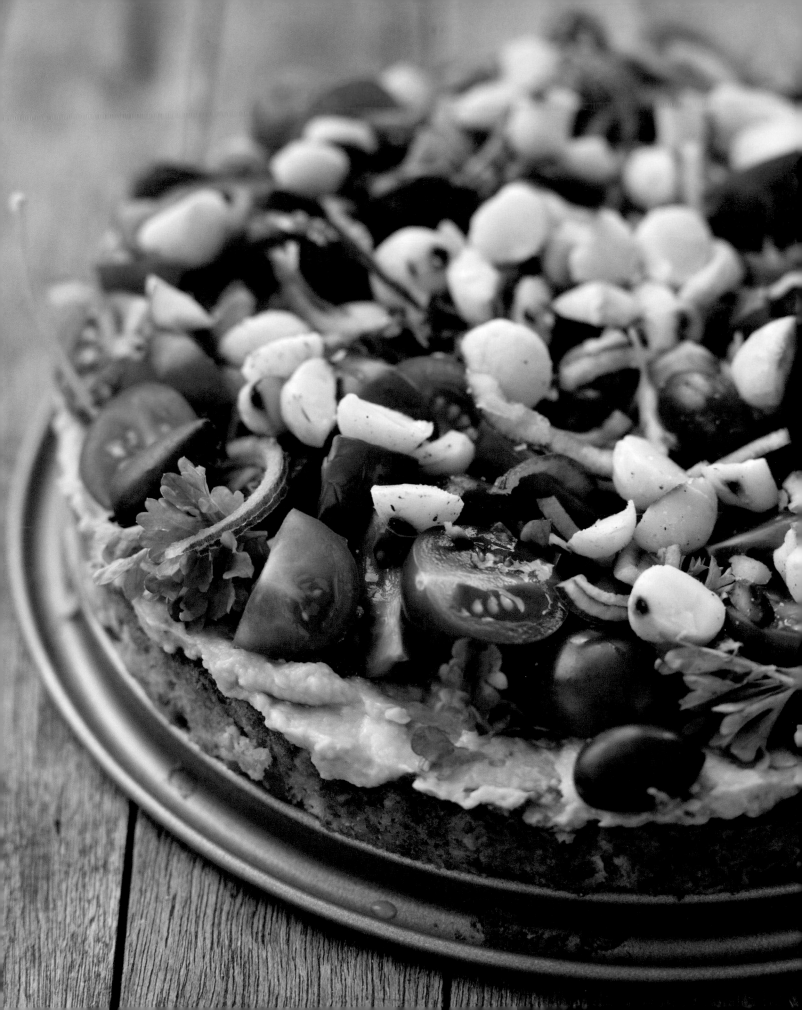

Sweet potato pie with guacamole and tomatoes

If you don't want to stick to raw food principles and bake the pie at a low temperature, you can use an oven and increase the temperature to 350 degrees (175 C). It should then be fully baked after about 45 minutes. You can also prepare and bake it the day or night before.

Pie

1 pie

1 sweet potato

2 carrots

1 red apple

1 ½ cups salted cashew nuts

Juice of ½ lemon

½ tsp salt

Guacamole

1 batch

½ red onion

1 ripe tomato

2 ripe avocados

½ pressed garlic clove

1 tbsp lemon juice

1–2 pinches cayenne

Salt and black pepper

Topping: tomatoes, arugula, sliced red onion, parsley, black olives, and roasted macadamia nuts

Preheat a dehydrator to 113 degrees (45 C), or see above for an alternative baking method. Peel and slice the sweet potato, carrots, and apple and place in a food processor with the nuts. Mix into a grainy mush, then add lemon juice and salt, mix a bit more, and pour into the pan. Bake for 7 hours in a springform pan lined on the bottom with parchment paper. Remove from oven and let cool.

Peel and chop the onion, tomato, and avocados. Place in a food processor with the garlic. Blend until the mixture achieves an even consistency, then add lemon juice, cayenne, salt, and pepper.

Spread a thick layer of guacamole over the chilled pie then top with the tomatoes, arugula, onion, parsley, olives, and macadamia nuts.

Macadamia pie with feta and broccoli

<u>4 small pies</u>
½ small zucchini
½ cup macadamia nuts
A pinch of sea salt

Filling
½ broccoli
Juice of ½ lemon
1 tbsp olive oil
1 carrot
4 small lettuce leaves
5 oz (150 g) feta cheese
1 tbsp olive oil
2 tbsp dried goji berries
1 tsp shelled hemp seeds
1 tsp oregano

Preheat a dehydrator to 113 degrees (45 C). Cut the zucchini into small pieces and place in a food processor with the nuts. Mix to a grainy dough and season with salt. Place the dough in 4 small springform pans. Bake in the dehydrator for about 4 hours.

Prepare the filling by chopping the broccoli into small florets and tossing them in lemon and oil. Peel and chop the carrot. Place a lettuce leaf in each pie dish and top with the lemon-marinated broccoli, carrot, and crumbled feta cheese. Drizzle some oil on top and sprinkle the goji berries, hemp seeds, and oregano on top.

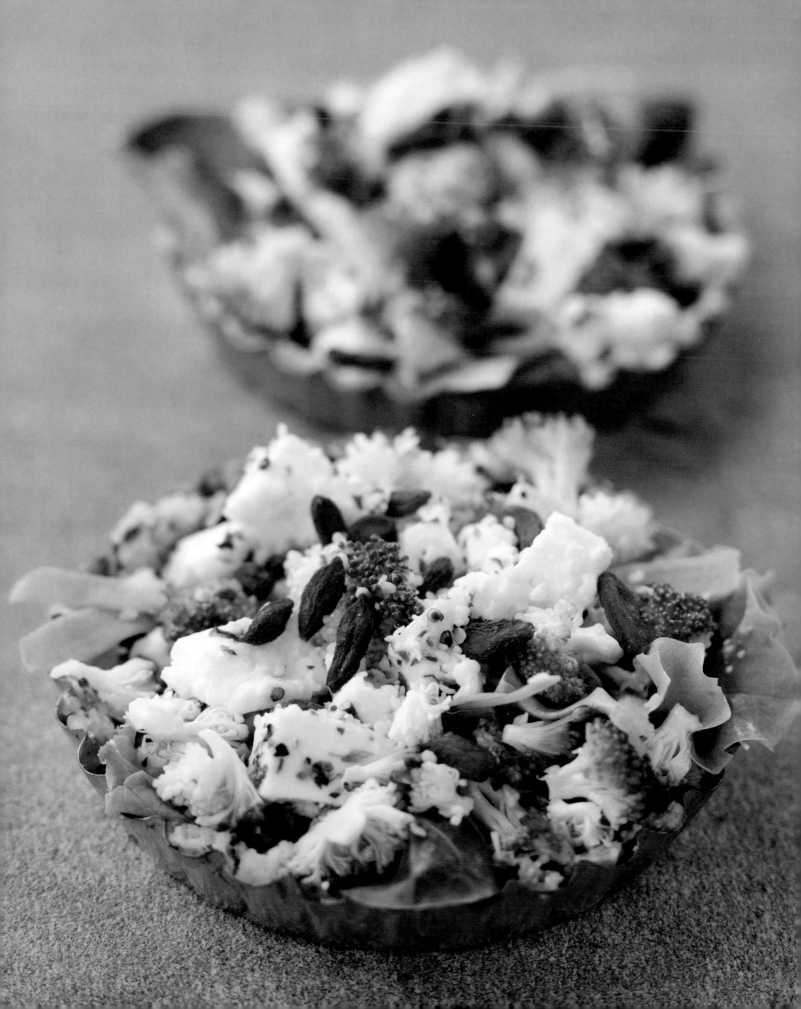

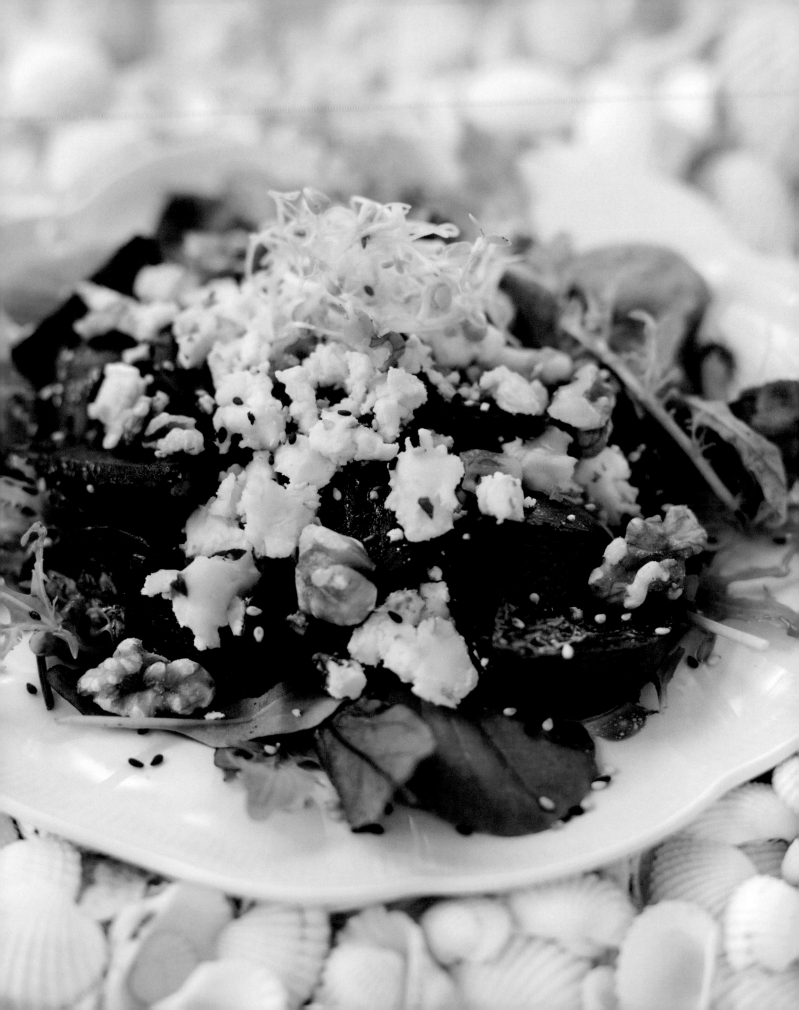

Marinated beets with feta cheese

<u>4 servings</u>

6 beets

2 tbsp olive oil

1 tbsp balsamic vinegar

1 tbsp honey

Salt and black pepper

1.7 oz (50 g) mixed lettuces

5 oz (150 g) feta cheese or goat cheese

½ cup (1 dl) sprouts

1.7 oz (50 g) walnuts

1 tbsp furikake

Boil the beets in lightly salted water for 30 minutes or until they become soft. Drain them and hold them under running cold water. Carve them into wedges. Blend oil, balsamic vinegar, honey, salt, and pepper in a bowl and add the beets. Stir it all together and let it sit for about 30 minutes or more. Arrange the lettuce on a plate and place the marinated beets on top. Top with feta cheese, sprouts, walnuts, and furikake.

Asian quinoa salad with coconut

<u>4 servings</u>

¾ cup (1 ½ dl) black quinoa

¾ cup (1 ½ dl) white quinoa

1 mango

2.5 oz (75 g) baby corn

2.5 oz (75 g) sugar snap peas

1 tbsp canola oil

1 grated garlic clove

2 tsp grated fresh ginger

1.7 oz (50 g) baby spinach

Juice of 1 lime

1 scallion

1.7 oz (50 g) cashews

¼ cup (½ dl) fresh sliced coconut

1 bunch coriander leaves, chopped

Boil the black and white quinoa separately according to the instructions on the packages (usually for about 13 minutes). Peel and slice the mango. Split the baby corn and sugar snaps down the middle. Heat a frying pan and add oil, garlic, and ginger. Sauté the corn and sugar snaps for a few minutes. Add the quinoa and let it all sauté for an additional minute or two. Place the spinach on plates and empty the quinoa salad on top. Drizzle the lime juice over the dish and top it off with chopped scallion, roasted cashews, coconut slices, and coriander.

WARM DISHES

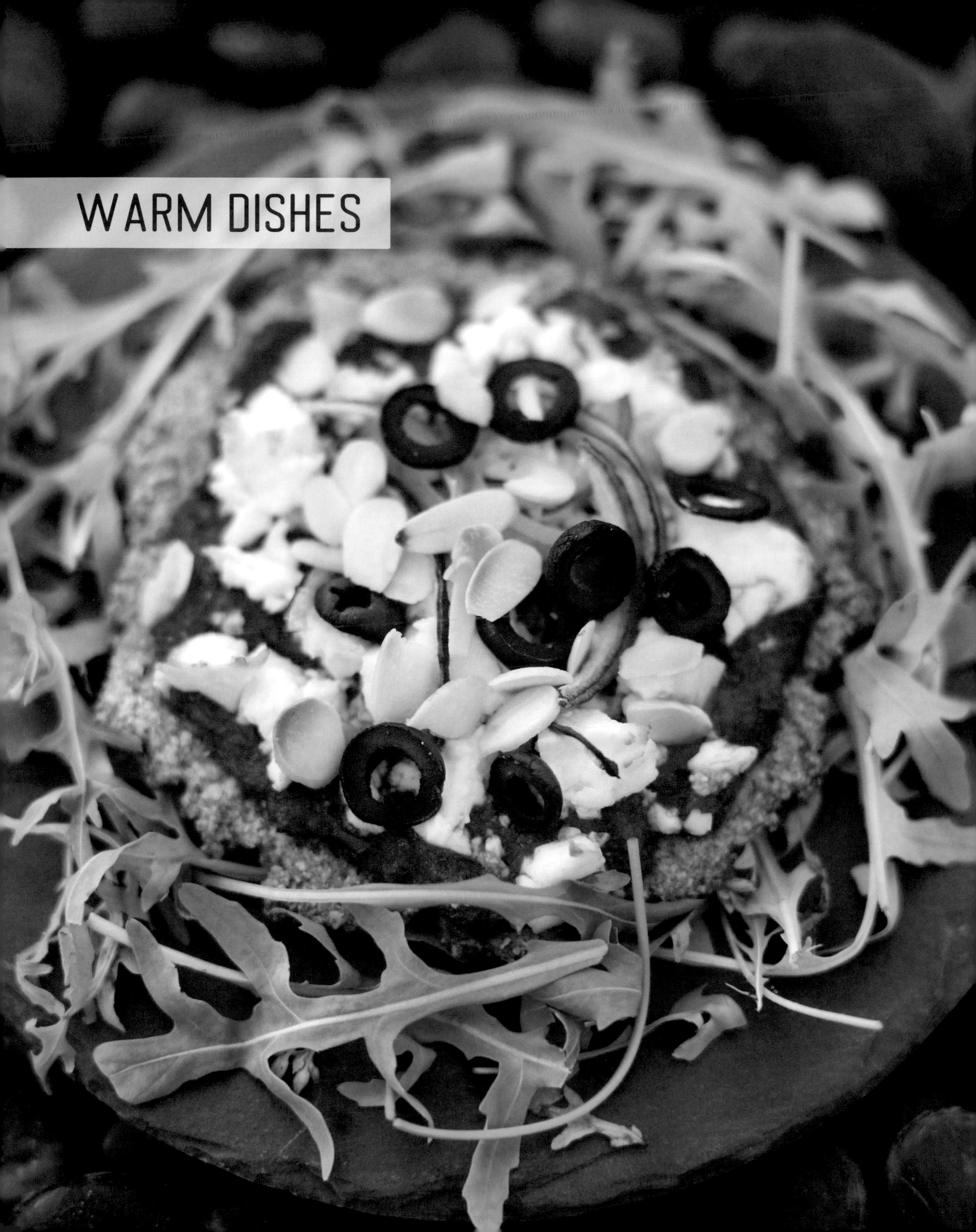

Pizza

4 small pizzas
Choose from three different toppings according to your taste preferences.

Pizza crust

7 oz (200 g) almonds
2 tsp psyllium husks*
½ tsp salt
½ tsp baking soda
¼ cup (½ dl) water
1 egg

*Psyllium husks are available for puchase online and at health-food stores.

Ajvar and feta cheese pizza

3.5 oz (100 g) feta cheese
1 red onion
10 black olives
1 cup (2 dl) ajvar relish
1 cup (2 dl) arugula
1 tbsp slivered almonds

Preheat the oven to 450 degrees (225 C). Grind the almonds into flour using a mortar and pestle. Mix the almond flour, psyllium husks, salt, and baking soda in a bowl. Add water and a beaten egg and mix until it achieves an even consistency. Let sit for 5 minutes. Roll the dough out into four round pieces on a parchment paper-lined baking sheet. Bake the crusts on the middle rack of the oven for about 10 minutes, or as instructed in the following recipes.

While the crusts bake, prepare one of the toppings.

Cut up the feta cheese. Peel and slice the onion and pit and chop the olives. When the crust is ready, spread the ajvar on it and add the feta cheese, onion, and olives. Sprinkle the slivered almonds on top and bake in the oven for 15 minutes. Top finished pizza with arugula and serve.

Beet and chèvre pizza

2 beets
½ cup (1 dl) arugula crème, p. 125
4 slices of chèvre cheese
1 tbsp honey
¼ cup (½ dl) walnuts
1 tsp thyme
1 cup spinach leaves

Peel and slice the beets. Spread a layer of arugula crème on the crust and place the beets and chèvre on top. Drizzle the pizza with honey and top with the walnuts and thyme. Bake on the middle rack of the oven for 15 minutes. Add the spinach leaves and serve.

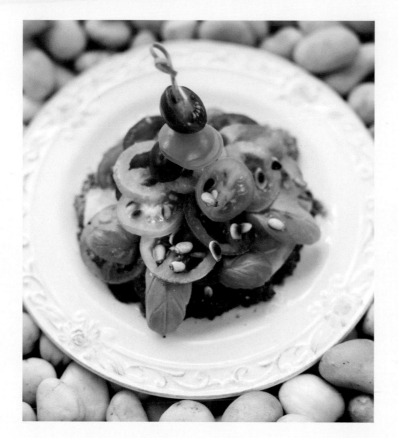

Tomato and pecorino pizza

¼ cup (½ dl) red pesto, p. 123
1.7 oz (50 g) pecorino cheese
8–9 oz (250 g) wild tomatoes
10 basil leaves
1.7 oz (50 g) pine nuts
Salt and pepper

Spread a thin layer of pesto over the crust. Slice the pecorino and distribute it evenly. Layer tomatoes and basil on top of the cheese. Roast the pine nuts in a dry frying pan for a few minutes, then sprinkle over the pizza and season with salt and pepper. Serve right away.

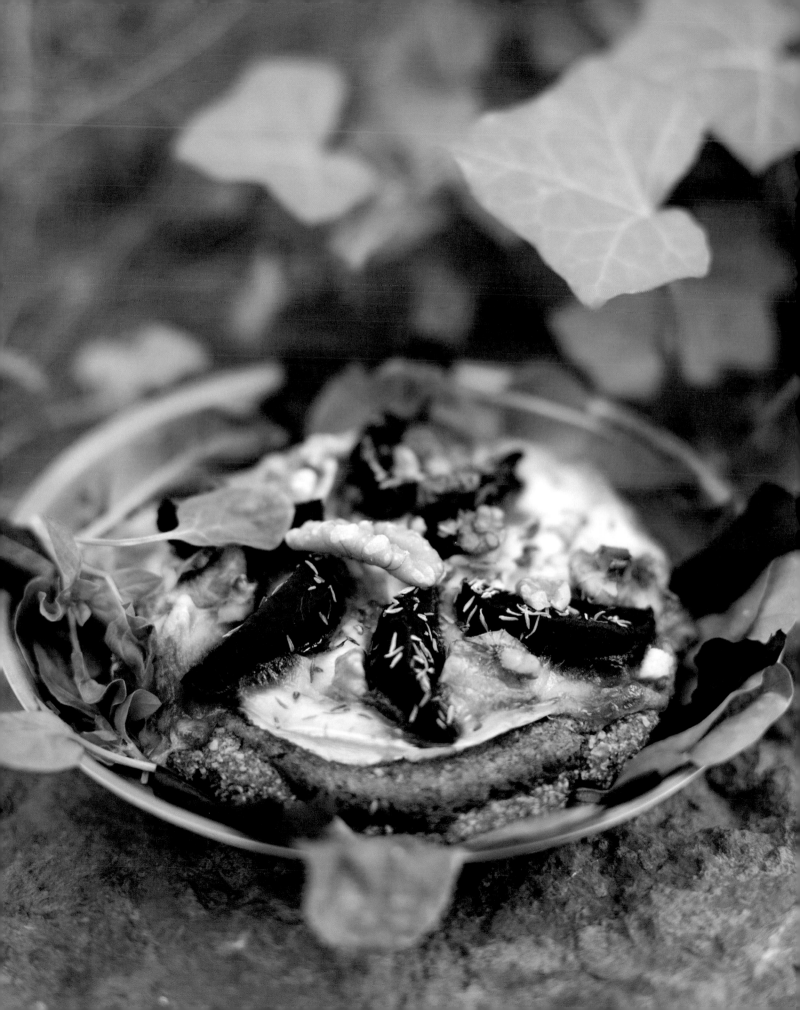

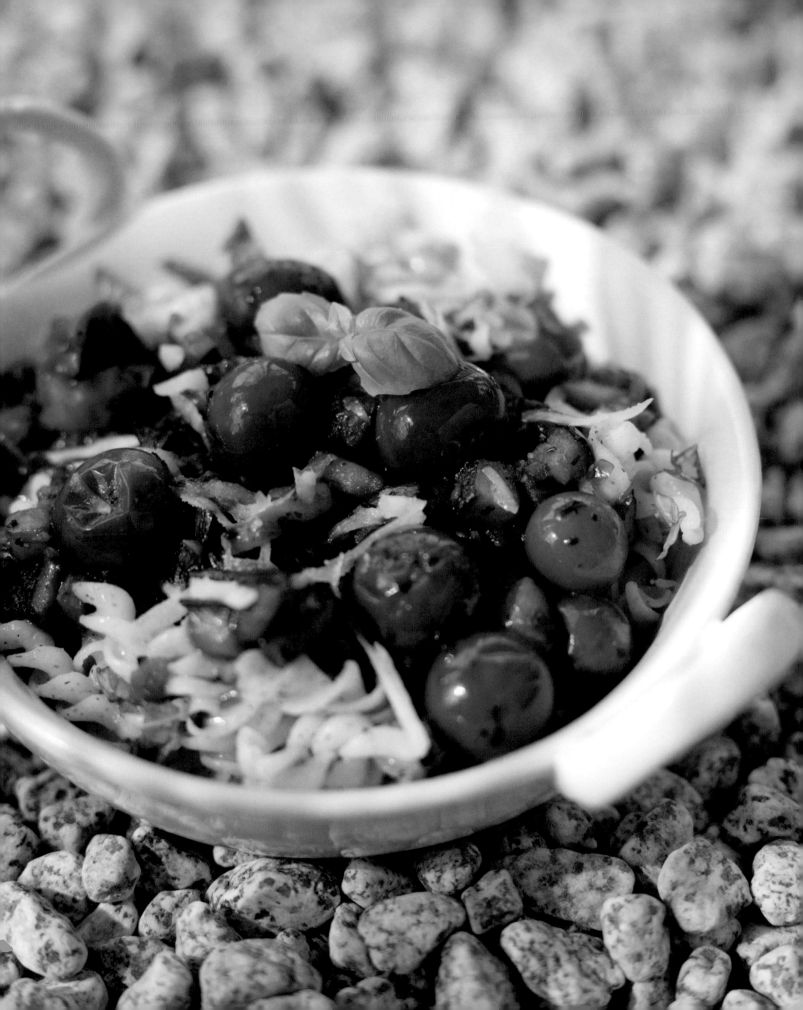

Buckwheat rotini with warm tomato sauce

4 servings

If you're craving pasta, there are a lot of good options that do not contain gluten or wheat. Many stores carry spaghetti, penne, and rotini made from buckwheat, rice, corn, or oats.

14 oz (400 g) buckwheat rotini (or a similar gluten- and wheat-free pasta)
½ yellow onion
½ red onion
2 garlic cloves
½ eggplant
½ zucchini
1 tbsp olive oil
5 sundried tomatoes
7 oz (200 g) cocktail or grape tomatoes
1 tsp dried basil
1 tsp dried oregano
20 black olives
¼ cup (½ dl) chopped fresh basil
Salt and black pepper
½ cup (1 dl) grated pecorino cheese

Boil the pasta as directed on the package. Peel and finely chop the onions and garlic. Dice the eggplant and squash. Heat the olive oil in a frying pan and sauté the onion, garlic, eggplant, and squash for a few minutes. Finely chop the sundried tomatoes. Add tomatoes, sundried tomatoes, basil, and oregano to the pan. Let simmer for about 10 minutes. Add the olives and the fresh basil. Season with salt and pepper. Serve the pasta with tomato sauce and top with grated pecorino cheese.

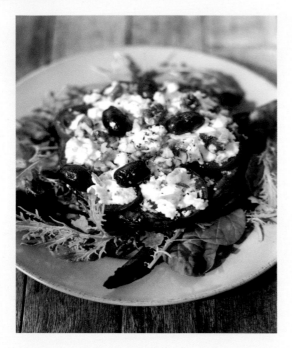

Baked portobello with feta cheese and tomato

<u>4 servings</u>
4 portobello mushrooms
2 tbsp olive oil
Salt and black pepper
½ batch tomato sauce, p. 83
3–4 tomatoes, sliced
5 oz (150 g) feta cheese
12–15 pitted black olives
1 oz (30 g) walnuts
1.7 oz (50 g) mixed salad

Preheat the oven to 400 degrees (200 C). Place the mushrooms on a baking pan and drizzle with olive oil. Add salt and pepper. Cover with tomato sauce and sliced tomatoes. Top with crumbled feta cheese, olives, and walnuts. Bake in the oven for about 20 minutes. Serve with mixed salad.

Falafel lettuce wraps

<u>4 servings</u>
2 cups (4 dl) boiled chickpeas, fresh or from a can
½ yellow onion
1 garlic clove
¼ cup (½ dl) chopped coriander or parsley
1 tsp cumin
Juice of ½ lemon
Salt and white pepper
½ cup (1 dl) millet seeds
¼ cup (½ dl) canola oil
8 cocktail tomatoes in various colors
1 red onion
1 head of lettuce
Banana pepper, parsley, and ajvar relish for topping

Rinse the canned chickpeas well. Peel and chop the yellow onion and garlic. Place the chickpeas, garlic, onion, coriander or parsley, and cumin in a food processor. Add the lemon juice and mix until it achieves an even consistency. Season with salt and pepper. Shape the mixture into balls and dredge them in the millet seeds. Heat the oil in a frying pan and panfry the falafel balls for about 5 minutes. Slice the tomatoes and red onion. Place the lettuce in four bowls and add the tomatoes, falafel, red onion, banana pepper, and parsley. Serve with ajvar relish if desired.

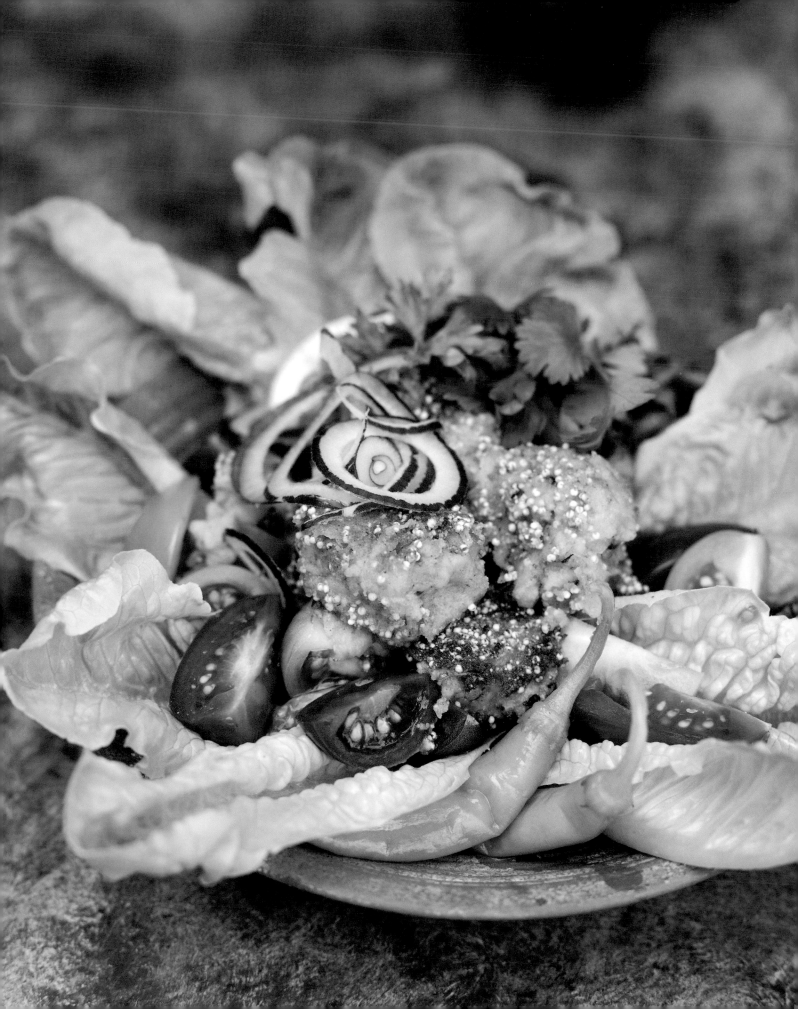

Rice noodles with coconut milk

4 servings

A tasty Asian sauce that's great with rice noodles or rice. Use organic coconut milk if possible, but it's not a must.

14 oz (400 g) rice noodles

2 carrots

1 yellow onion

2 garlic cloves

½–1 inch (2 cm) fresh ginger

1 tbsp canola oil

14.5 oz (1 small can) coconut milk

1 tsp powdered vegetable bouillon

2 tsp red curry paste

2 tsp honey

Juice of 1 lime

Salt and white pepper

1 head broccoli

5 oz (150 g) baby corn

2.5 oz (75 g) sugar snap peas

1 bunch coriander leaves, chopped

4 lime wedges and ¼ cup roasted cashews for garnish

Boil the rice noodles according to the instructions on the package (usually about 4–5 minutes). Peel and chop the carrots and onion. Grate the garlic and ginger. Heat a pot with canola oil and brown the carrots, onions, and garlic along with the ginger for a few minutes over medium heat. Add the coconut milk, bouillon, curry paste, honey, and lime juice. Season with salt and pepper. Let boil for about 5 minutes. Break the broccoli into florets and throw them in the pot with the baby corn and peas. Continue cooking for several minutes more. Serve with rice noodles, chopped coriander, lime wedges, and cashews.

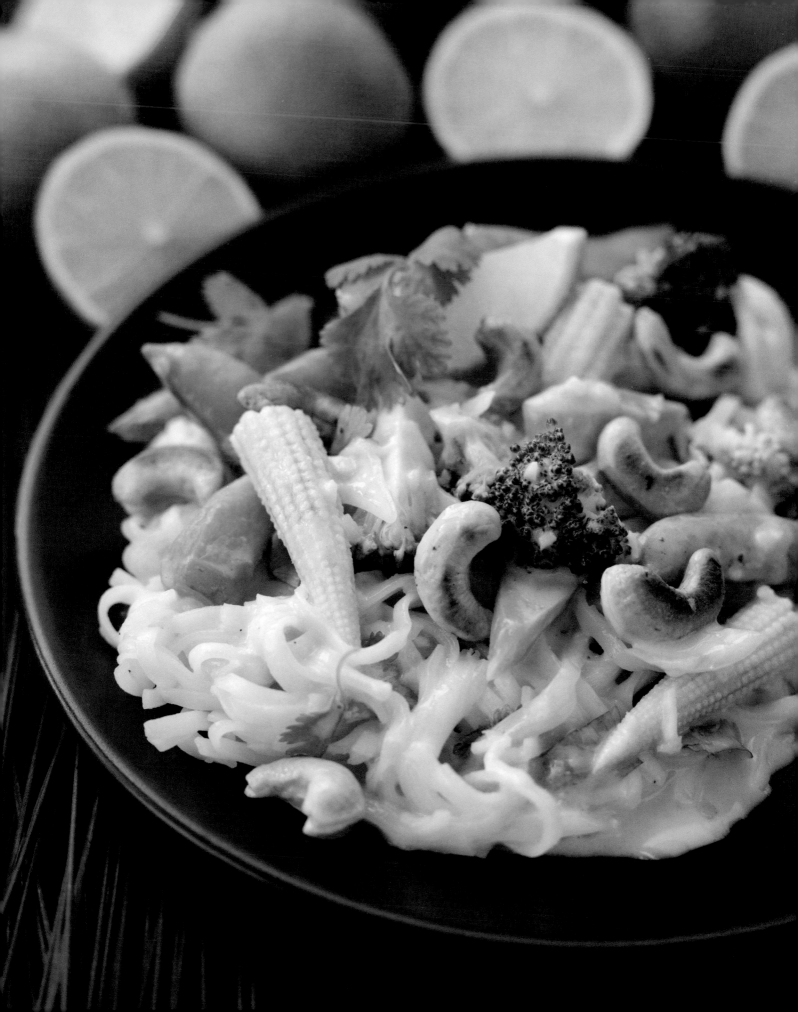

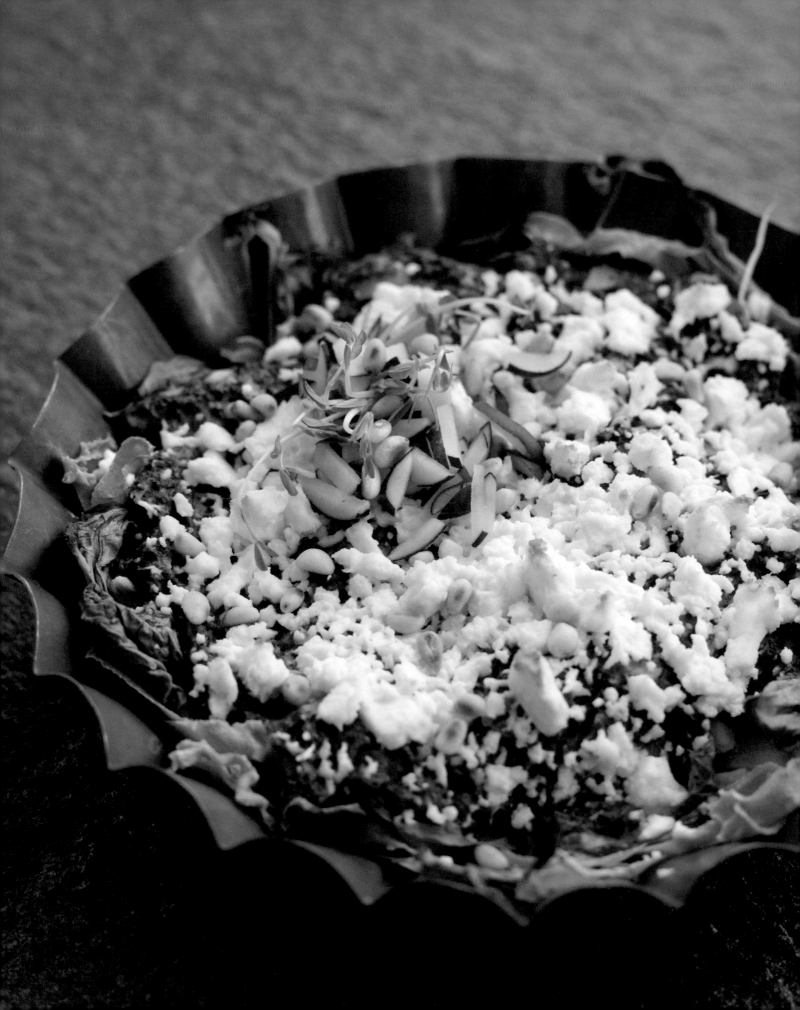

Spinach and feta casserole

4 servings

1 yellow onion

1 garlic clove

½ celery root

1 tbsp olive oil

10 oz (300 g) frozen spinach

½ cup (1 dl) soy-based heavy cream substitute (if you can't find this in stores, you can make your own)

Salt and black pepper

4 carrots

1 oz (30 g) fresh spinach leaves

5 oz (150 g) feta cheese

1.7 oz (50 g) pine nuts

Pea sprouts and radish for garnish

Preheat the oven to 400 degrees (200 C). Peel and finely chop the onion and garlic. Peel and chop the celery root. Heat a frying pan and sauté the onion, garlic, and celery root for a couple of minutes in oil. Add the spinach and heavy cream substitute. Let simmer for a couple of minutes. Season with salt and pepper. Peel and shave the carrots into paper-thin strips using a potato peeler. Cover the bottom of a baking dish with the strips and pour the spinach cream mixture over it. Cover with the fresh spinach leaves, then top with feta cheese and pine nuts. Bake in the oven for about 20 minutes. Garnish with some pea sprouts and chopped radishes.

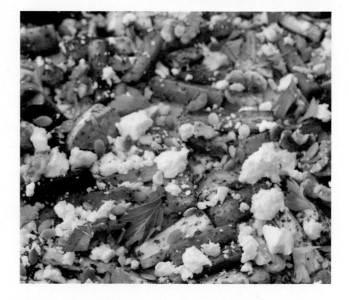

Roasted root vegetables with feta cheese

4 servings

3 carrots

2 parsnips

1 sweet potato

4 beets

2 tbsp olive oil

2 tsp balsamic vinegar

1 tbsp honey

1 tbsp mixed dried herbs (oregano, basil, thyme, etc.)

Salt and black pepper

5 oz (150 g) feta cheese

1.7 oz (50 g) walnuts

¼ cup (½ dl) pumpkin seeds

Preheat the oven to 440 degrees (225 C). Peel and chop the root vegetables into medium-sized pieces and spread them out on a baking sheet. Drizzle the vegetables with oil, vinegar, and honey and season with the herbs, salt, and pepper. Bake in the oven for about 20 minutes. Top with crumbled feta cheese, walnuts, and pumpkin seeds and serve.

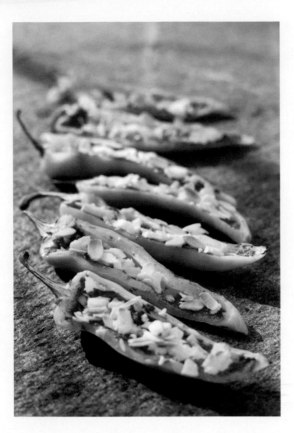

Stuffed rice leaves

<u>4 servings</u>

You should be able to find rice wrappers in the Asian section of your grocery store.

½ red onion
1 tbsp olive oil
1 cup (2 dl) cooked brown rice
2 tbsp chopped basil
Salt and black pepper
3 roasted bell peppers (from a jar)
8 rice wrappers
3.5 oz (100 g) feta cheese
Spinach leaves
Balsamic vinegar
Black sesame seeds

Side: Lettuce or pea sprouts

Preheat the oven to 400 degrees (200 C). Peel and finely chop the onion. Sauté the rice and onion for a few minutes in oil. Add basil and season with salt and pepper. Slice the bell peppers. Soak the rice wrappers (one at a time) for a few minutes. Place the bell peppers, feta cheese, spinach leaf, and rice mixture on the rice wrapper. Pour some balsamic vinegar on top and fold them into small packets. Sprinkle the packets with some sesame seeds and let them bake for about 15 minutes. Serve with a side of lettuce or pea sprouts.

Stuffed bell peppers

<u>4 servings</u>

As a variation, you can add red or green pesto or substitute goat cheese for feta if desired.

4 long yellow bell peppers
½ cup (1 dl) tapenade
5 oz (150 g) feta cheese
¼ cup (½ dl) slivered almonds
Lettuce for serving

Preheat the oven to 400 degrees (200 C). Slice the bell peppers in half and remove the core. Fill the halves with tapenade and feta cheese and top with slivered almonds. Bake for about 20 minutes. Serve with lettuce on the side.

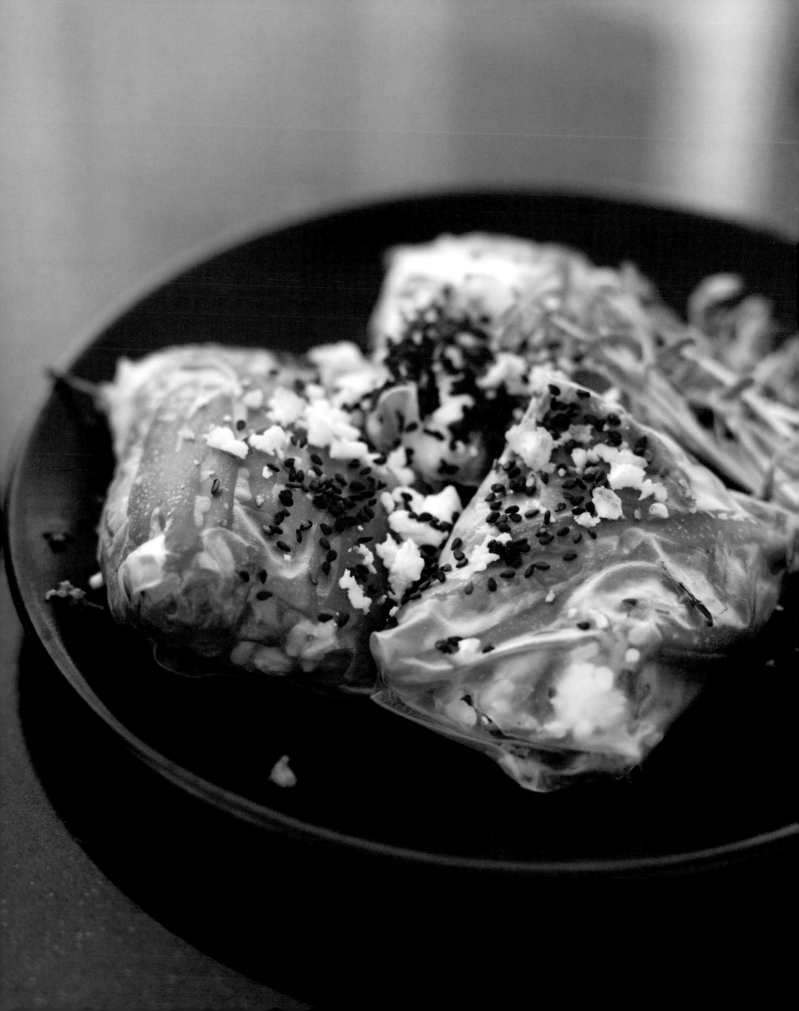

Mini eggplant, squash, and goat cheese towers with pine nut crust

4 servings (8 pieces)

1 eggplant

1 zucchini or summer squash

2 tbsp olive oil

1 tsp oregano

Salt and pepper

5 oz (150 g) goat cheese

2 red tomatoes

2 yellow tomatoes

Sage leaves for garnish

Pine nut crust

1.7 oz (50 g) pine nuts

1.7 oz (50 g) pecorino

½ garlic clove

Lemon juice

Salt and pepper

Preheat the oven to 440 degrees (225 C). Mix all ingredients for the crust in a blender or a food processor. Slice the eggplant into 16 slices and slice the squash into 8 slices. Fry the slices in oil for a couple of minutes on both sides. Season with oregano, salt, and pepper. Slice the cheese and tomatoes. Place 8 of the eggplant slices on a baking pan and cover with the pine nut mixture. Layer the squash, goat cheese, tomato, and eggplant on top and let bake for 10 minutes. Garnish with sage leaves.

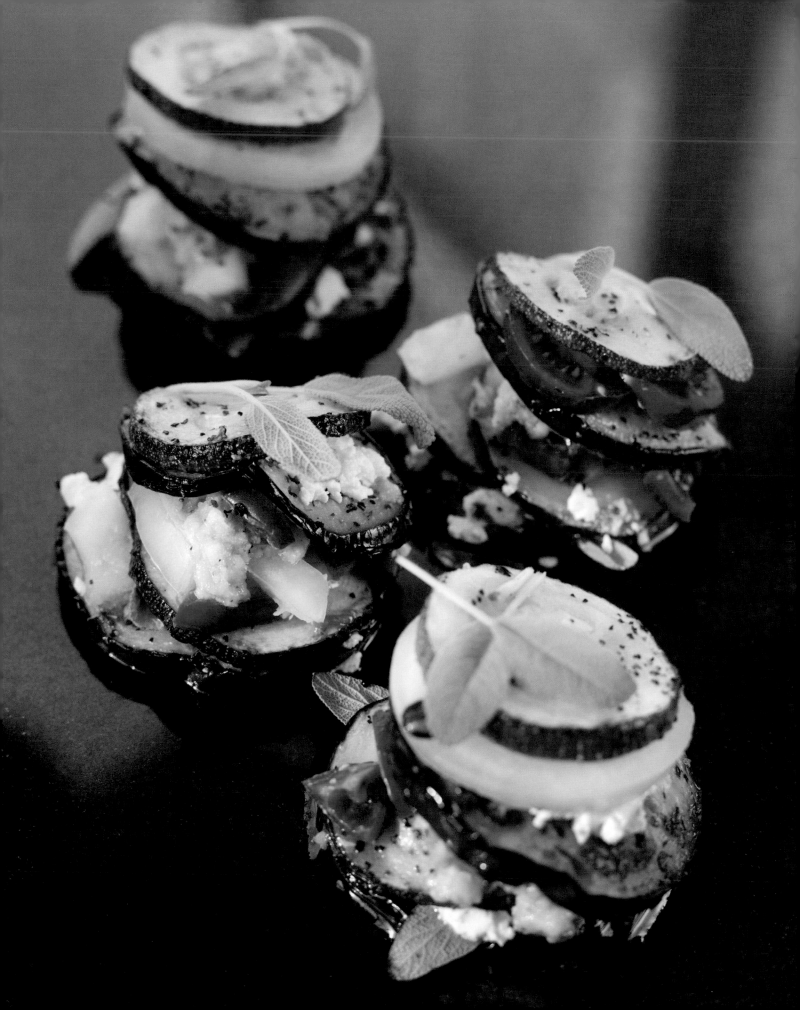

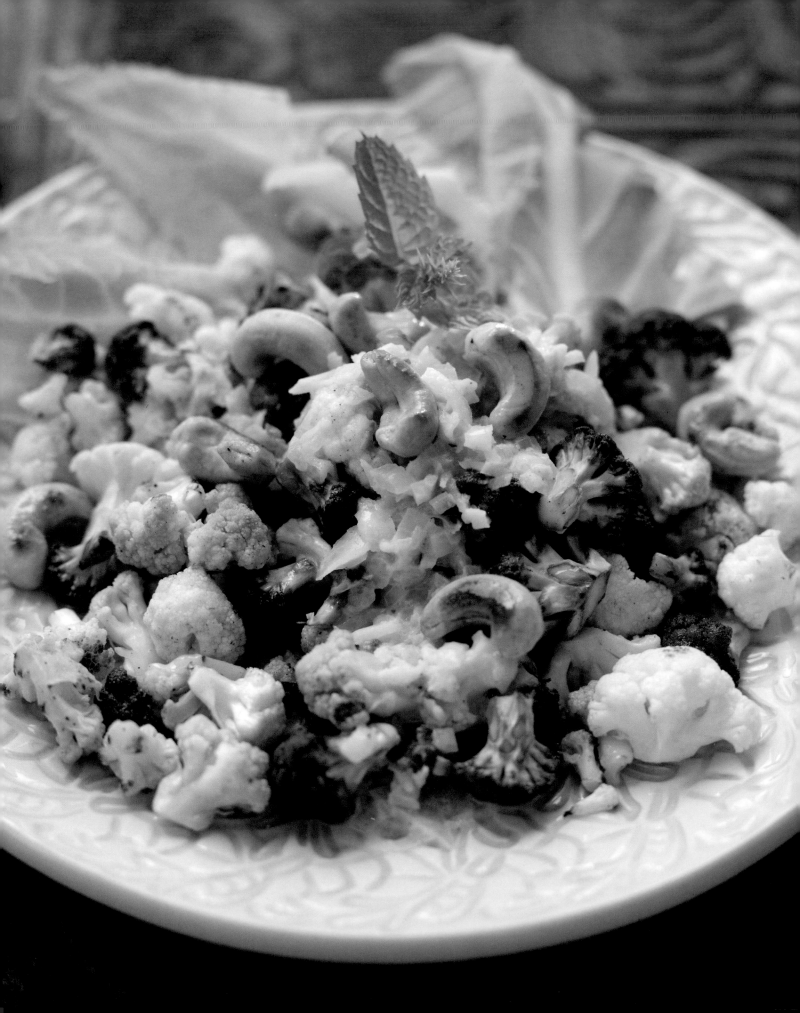

Tricolor cauliflower curry

<u>4 servings</u>
½ white cauliflower
⅓ purple cauliflower
⅓ green cauliflower
1 yellow onion
1 garlic clove
1 tbsp grated fresh ginger
1 tbsp canola oil
14.5 oz (1 small can) coconut milk
1 tbsp red curry paste
1 tbsp honey
Juice of 1 lime
Salt and white pepper
½ cup cashew nuts
1 head lettuce

Cut the cauliflower into small florets. Peel and finely chop the onion and garlic. Sauté the onion, garlic, and ginger in oil over medium heat for a couple of minutes. Add coconut milk, curry paste, honey, lime juice, salt, and white pepper and let it simmer for about 5 minutes. Add the cauliflower and continue cooking for a few minutes more. Roast the nuts in a dry frying pan. Plate the cauliflower curry, top with roasted nuts and lettuce, and serve.

Sliced eggplant with chèvre chaud

<u>4 servings</u>
1 eggplant
2 tbsp olive oil
Salt and pepper
8–9 oz (250 g) chèvre
1 tbsp white balsamic vinegar
2 tsp dried basil
3.5 oz (100 g) mixed lettuce
1 red bell pepper
1.7 oz (50 g) walnuts

Preheat the oven to 475 degrees (250 C). Cut the eggplant into 8 slices, about ½ inch (1 cm) thick each. Heat some oil in a skillet over medium heat and let the slices brown for a couple of minutes on each side. Season with salt and pepper. Place the eggplant slices side by side in two rows on a baking sheet. Cut the chèvre into 4 slices and place each slice so that it overlaps two slices of eggplant. Drizzle with balsamic vinegar and season with the dried basil. Bake for 5–7 minutes on the top rack of the oven. Rinse the lettuce and thinly slice the bell pepper. Arrange the lettuce and bell peppers on 4 plates to create beds for the eggplant. Chop the walnuts. Place the eggplant slices on top of the lettuce, sprinkle with the chopped walnuts, and serve.

SOUPS

Watermelon gazpacho

4 servings
A fresh and delicious soup that's served cold.

1 small watermelon
1 red onion
1 garlic clove
1 red chili
1 tbsp grated fresh ginger
Juice of 1 lemon
Salt and black pepper
4 celery stalks
1 cucumber
½ bunch of coriander

Remove the top of the watermelon and carve out the meat, keeping the rest of the rind intact (if the bottom end is rounded, cut away a small slice of the rind so that the watermelon can stand on end; you are creating a bowl). Peel and chop the onion and garlic. Cut the chili open, remove the core, and chop finely. Place the watermelon meat, onion, garlic, chili, and ginger in a food processor and blend until the mixture achieves a fairly even consistency. Add the lemon juice and season with salt and pepper. Pour the soup into the melon shell. Finely chop the celery and cucumber and add to the soup. Top with chopped coriander.

Creamy tomato soup with pumpkin seeds

4 servings
An appetizing cold soup.

4 tomatoes on the vine
2 garlic cloves
½ cup (1 dl) pumpkin seeds
1 bunch oregano
¼ cup (½ dl) olive oil
2 avocados
½ cup (1 dl) water
Salt and pepper

For topping: olive oil, 1 cup (2 dl) finely shredded carrots, and ½ cup (1 dl) raisins

Puree all of the ingredients except the water in a food processor until the mixture achieves an even consistency. Mix in water and season with salt and pepper. Pour into soup bowls or glasses. Drizzle with olive oil and top with shredded carrots and raisins.

Tomato soup with pesto-marinated feta cheese

4 servings

1 yellow onion

2 garlic gloves

1 tbsp olive oil

14.5 oz canned tomatoes (preferably whole and organic)

1 tbsp dried basil

1 vegetable bouillon cube

2 cups (5 dl) water

Salt and black pepper

Chili flakes

1 pint (or other small package) cherry tomatoes

5 oz (150 g) feta cheese

2 tbsp pesto

Peel and chop the onion and garlic. Heat some oil in a saucepan over medium heat and sauté the onion and garlic for a few minutes. Add the tomatoes, basil, bouillon cube, and water. Bring it to a boil and season with salt, pepper, and chili flakes. Pour into a food processor and blend, or use a hand blender. Pour the mixture back into the pot and bring to a boil again. Add more salt and pepper if needed. Add the cherry tomatoes and cook for a couple of minutes more. Chop the feta cheese and mix it with the pesto. Pour the soup in a bowl and top with the pesto-marinated feta cheese.

Spinach and broccoli soup with pecorino cheese

4 servings

4 cups (8 dl) water

1 tbsp vegetable stock

2 oz (50 g) frozen broccoli

2 oz (50 g) frozen spinach

3 shallots

1–2 garlic cloves

1 tbsp oil

Salt and black pepper

2 oz (50 g) fresh pecorino cheese

Boil water, stock, and broccoli in a pot for about 15 minutes. Add spinach and boil for an additional 5 minutes. Peel and chop the shallots and garlic. Sauté them in oil for a few minutes over medium heat, then add to the soup. Mix the soup in a food processor or using a hand blender and season with salt and pepper. Pour in a bowl. Grate or chop the cheese and sprinkle on top. Serve right away.

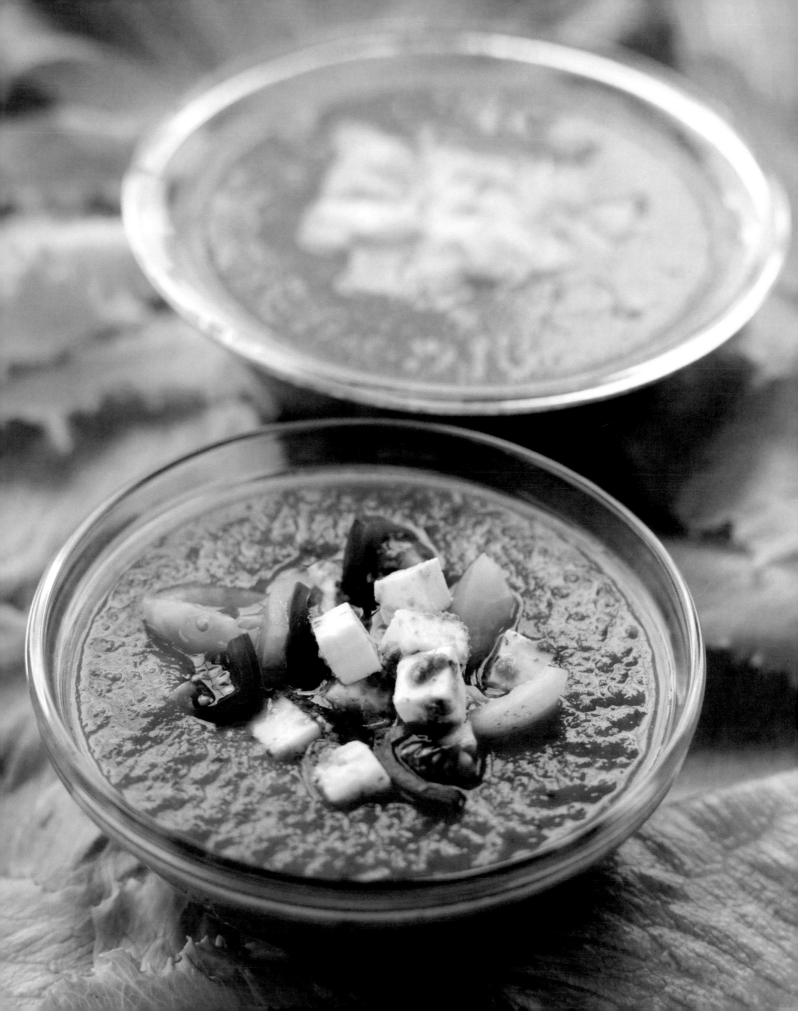

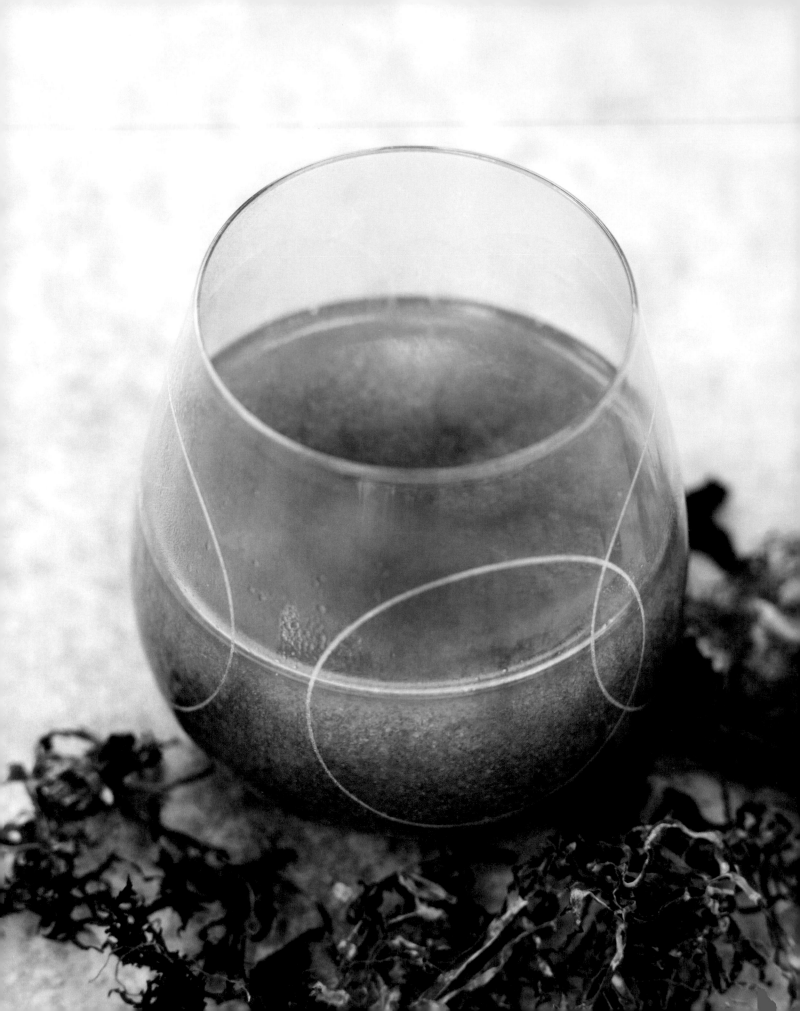

Miso soup

I will often have some miso soup to satisfy my hunger between meals, or just when I crave a little something. Miso is a Japanese soup that may be served in a variety of ways. You can easily make it from scratch at home. I usually buy portion-sized packets of miso powder and mix them with warm water. You can usually buy miso powder in grocery stores or at specialty health-food stores.

<u>1 serving</u>
1 cup (2 dl) water
1 portion bag of miso

Heat the water, mix in the miso powder, and enjoy.

Homemade rosehip soup

<u>1 batch</u>
1 cup (2 dl) dried rosehips or 2 cups (4 dl) fresh rosehips
5 cups (1 l) water (or more for a milder version)
1 stick vanilla
1 tsp lemon zest
4 dates
1 tbsp buckwheat or potato flour

Soak the rosehip in half of the water for about 10 minutes. Bring the rosehip water to a boil in a pot. Add the vanilla stick, lemon zest, and dates and let it boil for 5 minutes. Remove the vanilla stick and stir. Add the remaining water and thicken with the buckwheat or potato flour.

Raw power soup

<u>4 servings</u>
3 carrots
½ cucumber
8 tomatoes
2 red bell peppers
4 sundried tomatoes
½ small red onion, finely chopped
2 pitted dates
Black pepper
1 small chili, minced (optional)

Peel and dice the carrots and cucumber and set aside. Cut up the tomatoes and bell peppers and put them in a food processor. Add the sundried tomatoes, chopped red onion, and dates. Mix and season with pepper and chili, if desired. Place the carrots and cucumber in a bowl, pour the tomato soup on top, and serve.

Avocado and walnut soup

4 servings

A delicious and filling raw soup.

¾ cup (1 ½ dl) walnuts
2 avocados
1 garlic clove
4 sundried tomatoes in oil
1 tbsp chopped dill
½ cup (1 dl) olive oil
Juice of ½ lemon, freshly squeezed
2 cups (4 dl) water

For garnish:
¼ cup (½ dl) chopped walnuts
1 avocado, diced
Chopped dill

Soak the ¾ cup of the walnuts overnight. Drain them and put them in a food processor. Add the 2 avocados, peeled, pitted, and chopped, along with the garlic, sundried tomatoes, and tablespoon of dill. While the ingredients are being mixed add the olive oil and freshly squeezed lemon juice. Add water as needed to give the soup a fluid consistency. Pour in a bowl and top it off with the remaining walnuts, avocado, and dill.

Chantarelle soup with rice noodles

4 servings

1 tbsp canola oil
5 cups (1 l) fresh chanterelles (or 1 cup/2 dl dried)
1 red chili
1 yellow onion
Salt and white pepper
5 cups (1 l) water
1 tbsp bouillon (powdered)
4 oz (125 g) rice noodles
5 oz (150 g) sugar snap peas
1 tbsp fish sauce
1 cup (2 dl) chives, cut lengthwise into strips

Sauté the mushrooms for 10 minutes in oil over medium heat. Finely chop the chili and slice the onion and sauté with the mushrooms for a couple of minutes. Season with salt and white pepper. Boil water and bouillon in a pot. Add the rice noodles and cook for 2–3 minutes. Slice the sugar snaps. Add fish sauce, mushrooms mixture, chives, and sugar snap peas. Return to a boil and serve right away.

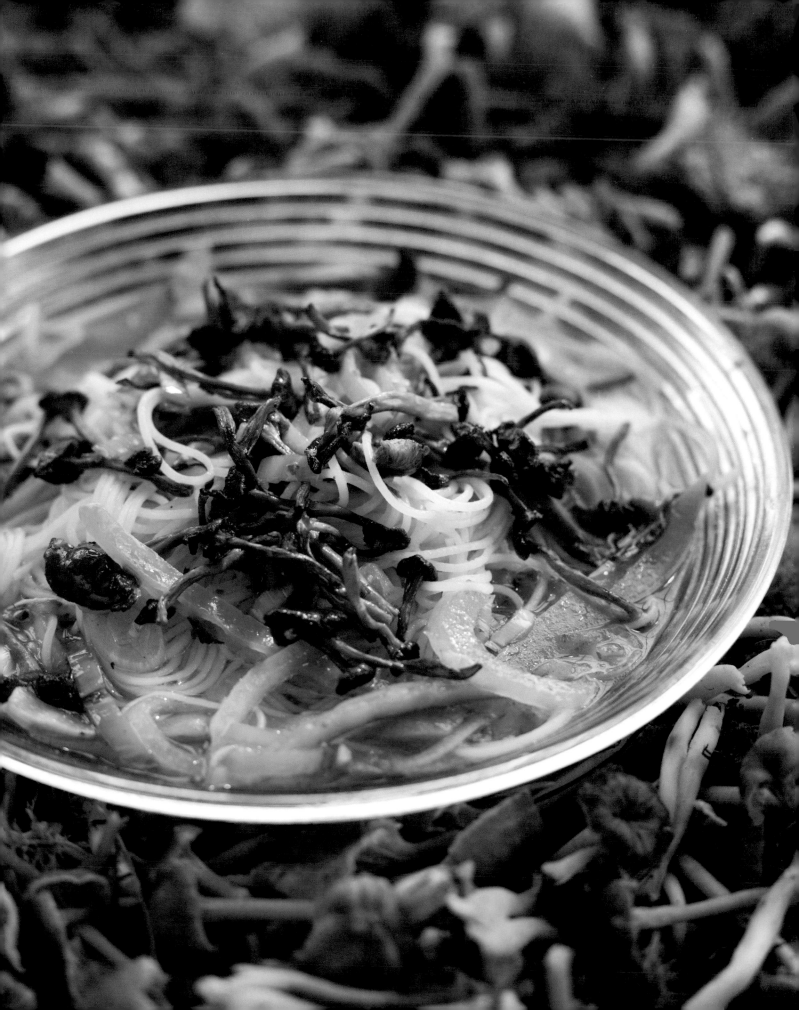

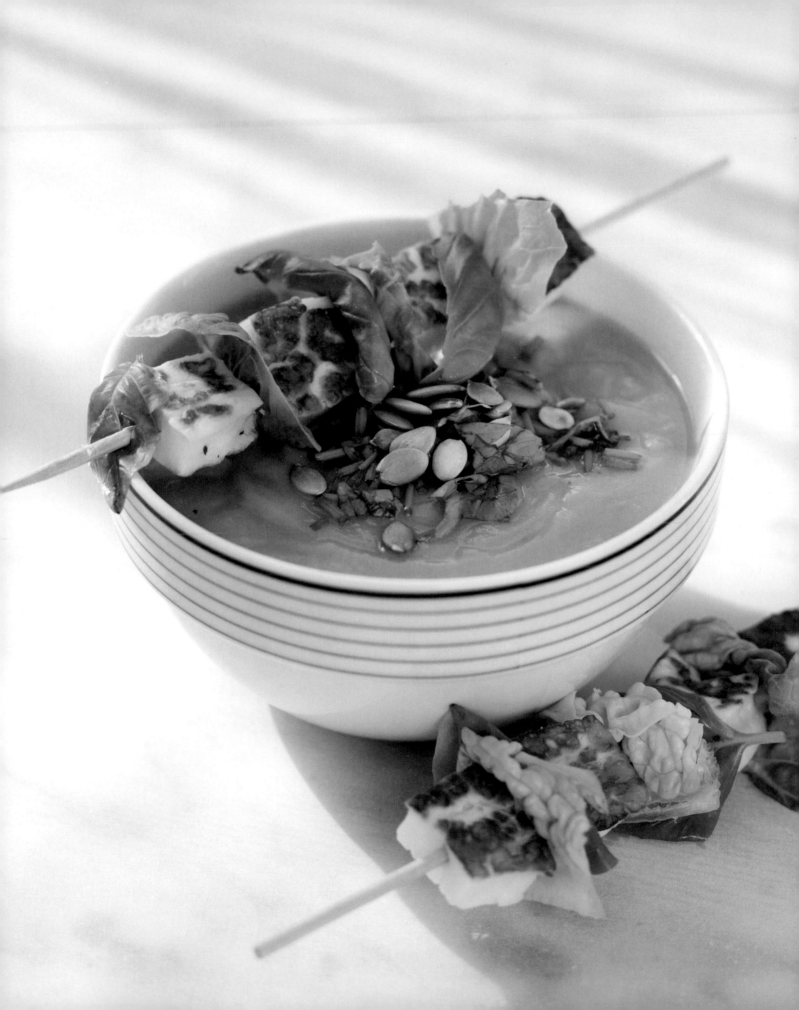

Sweet potato soup
with halloumi skewers

4 servings
4 small sweet potatoes
1 yellow onion
1 garlic clove
Olive oil for frying
1 tbsp bouillon
5 cups (1 l) water
Salt and white pepper

For garnish:
¼ cup (½ dl) mixed herbs (basil, chives, etc.)
2 tbsp pumpkin seeds

Halloumi skewers
8 skewers, 2 per serving
3 oz (85 g) halloumi cheese
2 leaves romaine lettuce
Olive oil for frying
Basil
8 wooden skewers

Peel and chop the potatoes, onion, and garlic. Heat a little oil in a pot over medium heat and sauté the onion and garlic for a few minutes. Add bouillon, water, and potatoes. Let it boil for about 20 minutes. Mix the soup in a food processor or using a hand blender. Add more water if needed. Return the soup to the pot and bring to a boil. Season with salt and white pepper.

Cut the cheese into bite-sized pieces and cut up the lettuce leaves. Heat some oil in a frying pan, then brown the cheese on both sides. Stick the cheese, lettuce bits, and basil on the skewers. Distribute the soup in bowls and top with herbs and pumpkin seeds. Serve with the halloumi skewers.

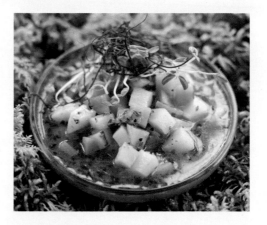

Root vegetable soup
with saffron

4 servings
2 carrots
2 parsnips
½ small celery root
1 garlic clove
½ yellow onion
1 tbsp olive oil
¼ tsp saffron
1 tbsp powdered bouillon
5 cups (1 dl) water
Salt and black pepper
1 tsp dried oregano
Sprouts (pea sprouts or similar)

Peel and cube the carrots, parsnips, and celery root. Finely chop the garlic and onion. Heat some oil in a pot and sauté the vegetables for a couple of minutes, then add the saffron. Add the bouillon and water. Let it boil for about 15 minutes. Season with salt, black pepper, and oregano. Garnish with the sprouts.

Roasted bell pepper soup with cress and goji berries

<u>4 servings</u>

4 red bell peppers

1 yellow onion

1 garlic clove

4 yellow tomatoes

1 tbsp olive oil

2 ½ cups (5 dl) water

1 tbsp bouillon (powdered)

Salt and black pepper

Goji berries and cut cress for garnish

Preheat the oven to 475 degrees (250 C). Cut the peppers in half and remove the cores. Place them face down on an oiled baking sheet and bake until they are soft and have some color. Peel off the skin. Peel and chop onion and garlic. Cut up the tomatoes and roasted bell peppers. Heat some oil in a saucepan over medium heat and sauté the onion and garlic for few minutes. Add the tomatoes and peppers and continue cooking for a couple of minutes. Add the water and bouillon. Let it boil for 5 minutes. Mix the soup with a hand blender and season with salt and pepper. Pour in a bowl and top with goji berries and cress.

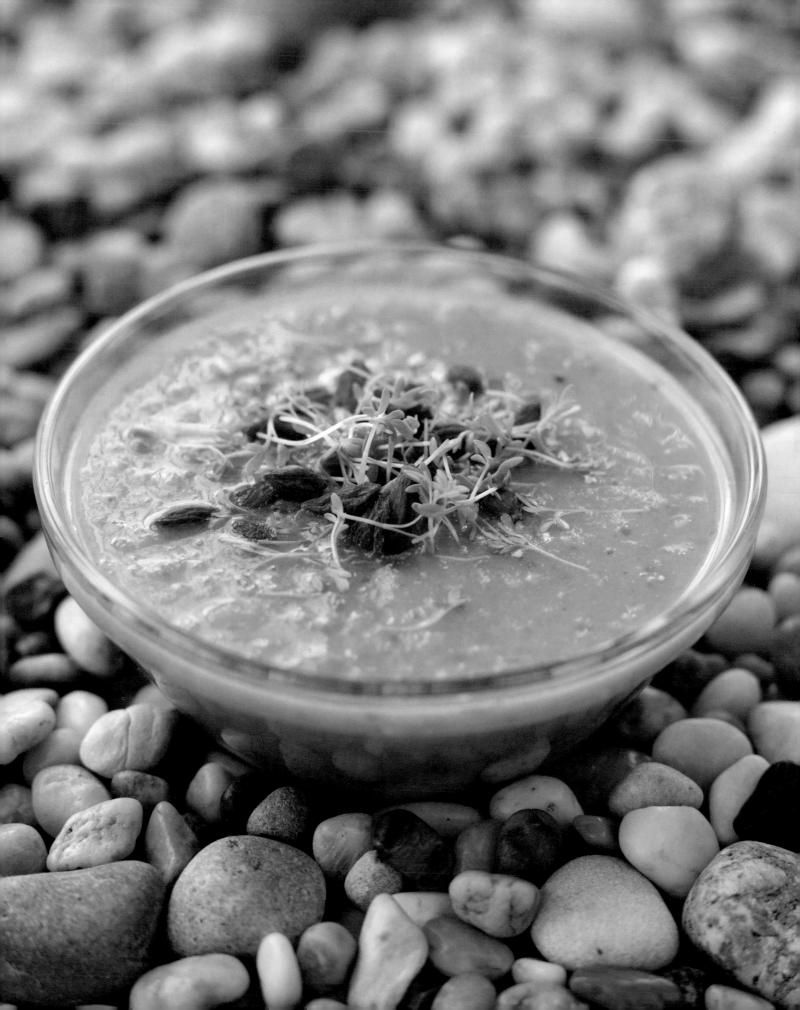

DESSERTS & SWEETS

Mixed melon dessert

4 servings

For this dessert fruit salad, choose seasonal berries and fruits or use whatever you have lying around the kitchen.

4 cantaloupes
½ watermelon
1 orange
1 clementine
4 apricots
½ cup (1 dl) raspberries
½ cup (1 dl) blueberries
4 currant clusters
Juice of 1 lemon
Juice of 1 lime

Cut off the tops of the cantaloupes and watermelon, and dig out the meat using a spoon or melon scoop. Peel and slice the orange and clementine. Cut the apricots into small pieces. Distribute the different fruits evenly among the four cantaloupe bowls. Squeeze lime and lemon juice over the fruit and serve.

Cloudberry "ice cream" with cacao nibs

4 servings

If you can't find cloudberries in your area, substitute with raspberries or blackberries for a delicious alternative.

3 frozen bananas
8–9 oz (250 g) frozen cloudberries
2 tbsp cacao nibs

Mix the banana and cloudberries into an "ice cream" using a food processor. Place in glasses and top with the cacao nibs. Serve right away.

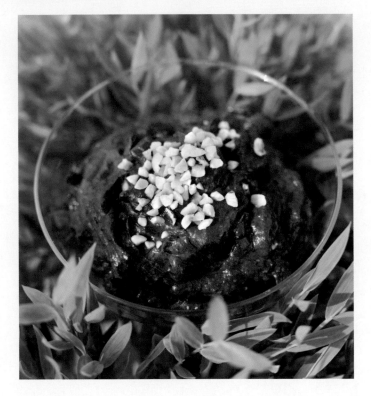

Avocado and chocolate mousse

<u>4 servings</u>
A deliciously creamy raw-food mousse.

½ cup (1 dl) dried dates
2 avocados
½ cup (1 dl) water
4 tbsp honey
1 tsp vanilla powder
1 tsp cocoa powder
¼ cup (½ dl) chopped hazelnuts

Soak the dates in water for 30 minutes. Peel and cut up the avocados, removing the pit, and place in a food processor. Add dates, water, honey, vanilla, and cocoa and let it mix until it achieves an even, creamy consistency. Serve in a tall glass. Top with chopped hazelnuts.

Lime-and-mint-marinated fruit

<u>4 servings</u>
The Pakistani mango is yellower and longer than a regular mango. It is also a lot sweeter and juicier. Try it once and you will never go back!

2 Pakistani mangoes
4 peaches
2 ½ cups (1 l) strawberries
2 limes
½ bunch mint leaves
2 tbsp honey

Peel and cut the mangoes and peaches into small pieces. Place them in a bowl. Rinse and slice the strawberries. Rinse the lime carefully and grate the peel. Mix the grated lime peel with the rest of the fruit and squeeze the juice on top. Chop the mint and mix with the fruits. Drizzle with honey and serve.

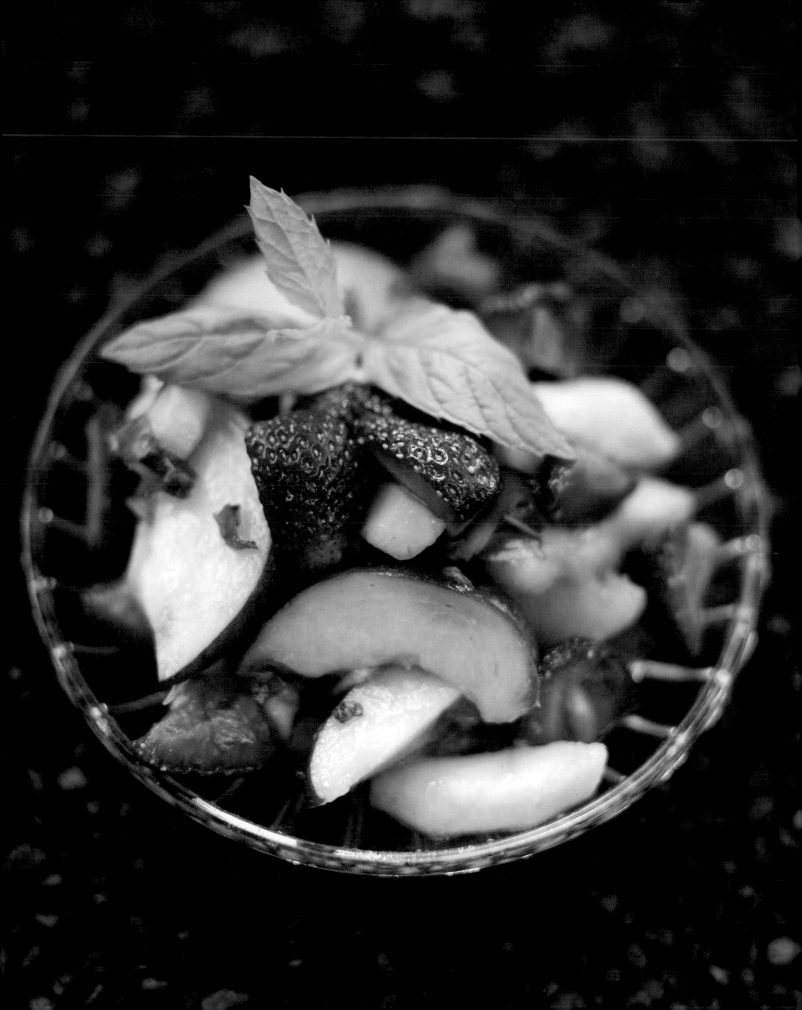

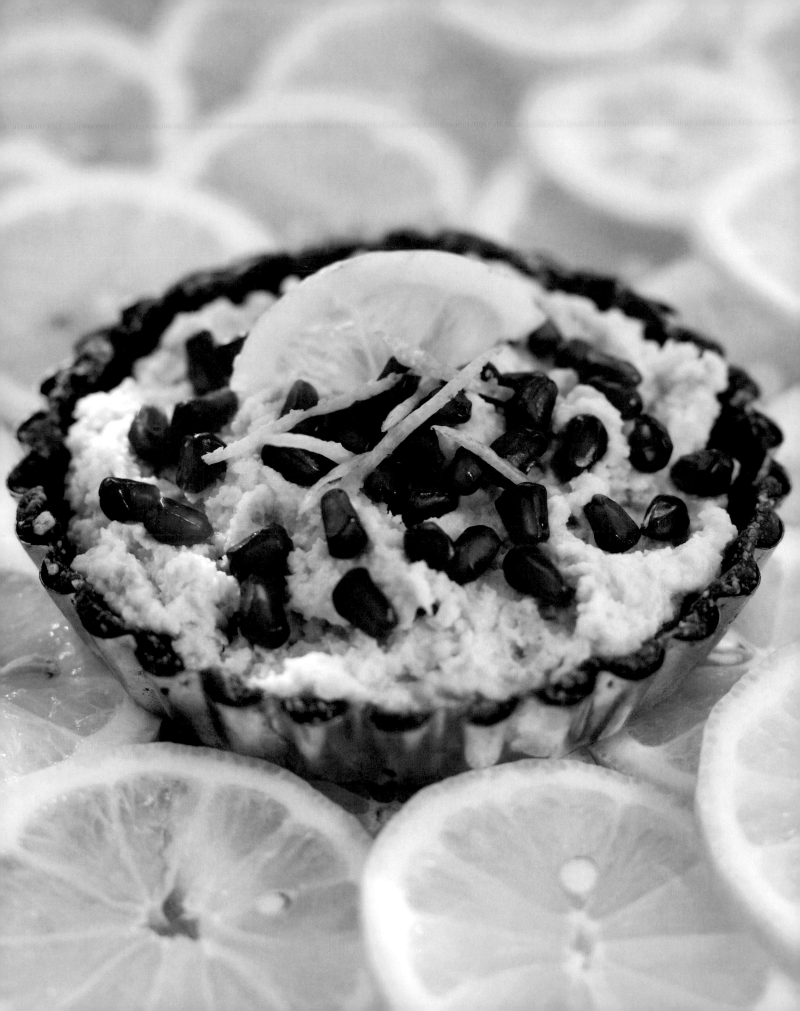

Lemon tart with pomegranate

4 servings

Crust
1 ½ cups (3 dl) cashews
4 dried apricots
2 tbsp honey
Grated peel of ½ orange
1 tbsp cocoa

Filling
1 ½ cups (3 dl) cashews
½ cup (1 dl) water
¼ cup (½ dl) mango, cut into pieces
Zest and juice of 1 lemon

1 pomegranate and 1 grated lemon peel for garnish

Place all the ingredients for the crust in a food processor and mix. Roll out and place the dough in a small (6 in, or 15 cm) spring-form pan, shaping it to form a pie shell. Refrigerate for 30 minutes.

Put the cashews, water, mango, lemon juice, and lemon zest in the food processor and mix until it becomes a fluffy cream. Pour the finished cream into the shell and garnish with pomegranate and lemon zest.

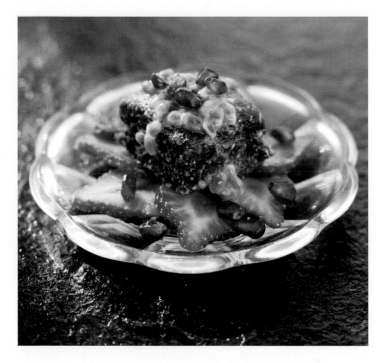

Fudge with passion fruit

4 servings
4 dried figs
2 passion fruit
1 ½ cups (3 dl) cashews
2 tbsp honey
1 tbsp cocoa

Fro garnish: 8 strawberries, 2 passion fruits, and ½ pomegranate

Soak the figs in water for 30 minutes, then drain. Cut the passion fruit in half, scoop out the insides, and place in a food processor. Add the fig and the remaining ingredients. Blend until it achieves a thick and even consistency. Shape into a square on a plate, cover with saran wrap, and let it chill in the refrigerator for an hour. When it is done, cut the fudge into four pieces.

Slice the strawberries and the passion fruit. Arrange the strawberry slices on a plate and place the fudge on top. Garnish with the passion fruit and pomegranate seeds and serve.

Almond muffins with blueberries and mango

6–8 Muffins

Vanilla powder doesn't contain any additives or sugars. It is a completely natural flavor component and it tastes wonderful.

2 oz (50 g) dried mango
7 oz (200 g) almonds
3.5 oz (100 g) brazil nuts
¼ cup (½ dl) water
¼ cup (½ dl) honey
1 tsp vanilla powder
1 tsp baking powder
2.5 oz (70 g) blueberries
4 eggs

2 slices of dried mango and ¼ cup (½ dl) of blueberries for topping

Preheat the oven to 400 degrees (200 C). Place muffin cups in the muffin tin. Soak the mango in water for a few minutes. Pulverize the almonds in a food processor and pour the resulting flour in a bowl. Put the Brazil nuts, mango, and water in the food processor and blend for a little while before you add the almond flour. Add honey, vanilla powder, baking powder, and 2.5 oz (70 g) of the blueberries. Whisk the eggs and add to the mixture. Scoop the batter into the muffin cups, filling them halfway. Shred the dried mango finely with a sharp knife and place on top of the muffins along with the remaining blueberries. Bake on the middle rack of the oven for 25 minutes.

Almond muffins with apple and cinnamon

6–8 Muffins
10 oz (300 g) almonds
1 cup (2 dl) dried apple rings, cut into pieces
1 tsp cinnamon
1 tsp cardamom
1 tsp baking soda
½ cup (1 dl) dried coconut, shredded and unsweetened
½ cup (1 dl) honey
4 eggs

For topping:
¼ cup (½ dl) slivered almonds
¼ cup (½ dl) dried apple rings, cut into pieces

Preheat the oven to 400 degrees (200 C). Place muffin cups in the muffin tin. Pulverize the almonds using a food processor. Pour the almond flour into a bowl and add the 1 cup of cut-up apple rings, cinnamon, cardamom, baking soda, coconut, and honey. Whisk the eggs and add to the batter. Spoon the batter into the muffin cups, filling them halfway. Top with slivered almonds and remaining dried apple rings. Bake on the middle rack of the oven for 25 minutes.

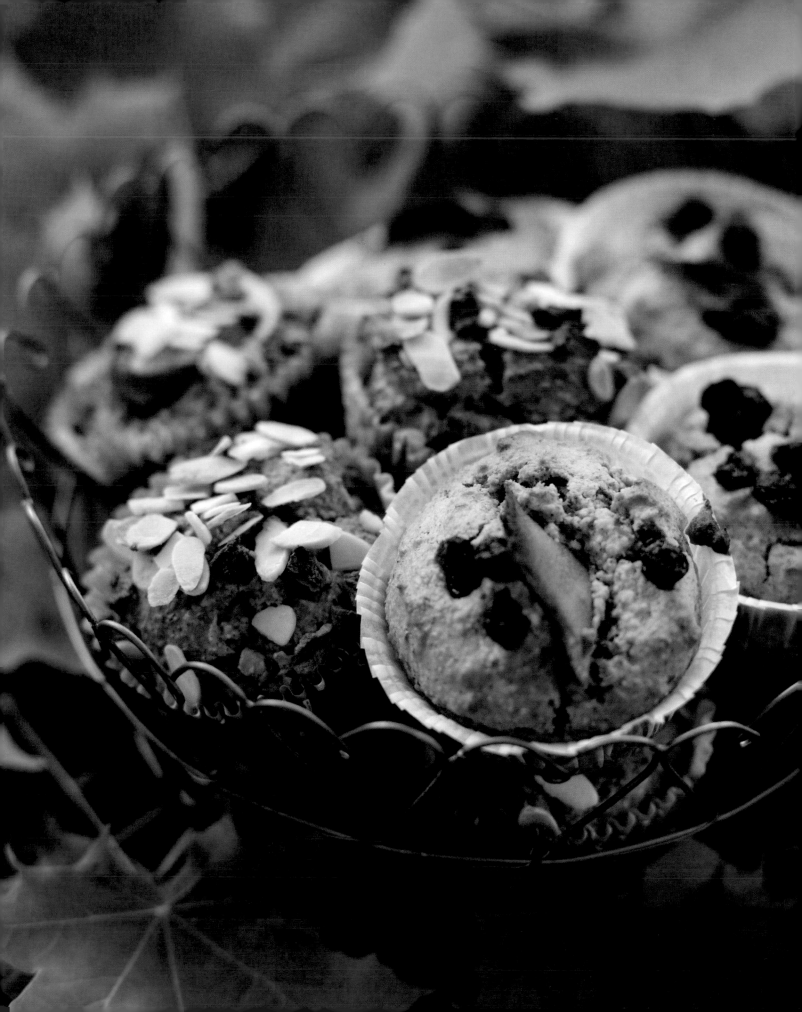

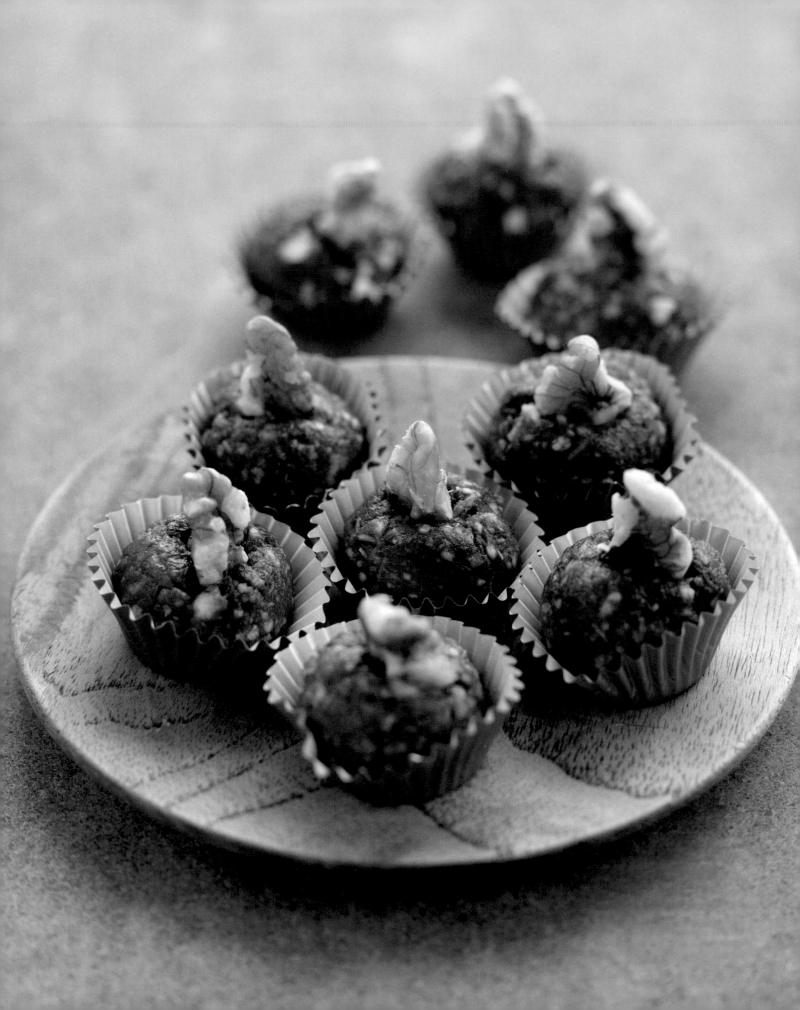

Walnut and chocolate truffles

about 12 balls
1 cup walnuts
½ cup cashews
5 dates
2 tbsp coconut fat
1–2 tbsp cocoa
Water, as needed
Walnuts for topping

Mix all ingredients in a food processor. Add water if necessary. Shape the mixture into balls and place them in mini muffin cups. Top with walnuts. Keep in the refrigerator or freezer.

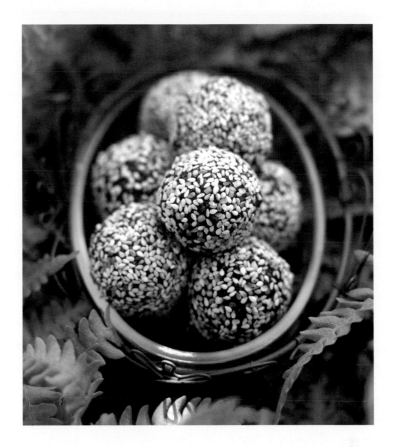

Mint truffles

About 15 balls
2 ½ cups (5 dl) cashews
¼ cup (½ dl) honey
7 drops of peppermint oil
¼ cup (½ dl) cocoa
½ cup (1 dl) roasted coconut flakes

Pulverize the cashews into flour using a food processor. Add honey, peppermint oil, and cocoa and mix until you have an even dough. Shape the dough into balls and dredge them in the coconut flakes. Keep in the refrigerator or freezer.

Spirulina balls

About 12 large balls
½ cup (1 dl) sunflower seeds
½ cup (1 dl) pumpkin seeds
½ cup (1 dl) cashews, unsalted
2 tsp spirulina powder
¼ cup (½ dl) raisins
5 dried apricots
1 tbsp honey
¼ cup (½ dl) sesame seeds

Mix all of the ingredients except the sesame seeds in a food processor until you have an even dough. Shape the dough into balls and dredge them in the sesame seeds. Keep in the refrigerator or freezer.

Banana mousse with chocolate and roasted coconut

<u>4 servings</u>
3 frozen bananas
1 tbsp cocoa
1 tbsp honey
1 tbsp water

Topping:
2 tbsp chopped pistachio nuts
2 tbsp roasted coconut flakes

Mix all of the ingredients in a food processor. Place the mousse in bowls and top with pistachios and coconut.

Plum pie

<u>8 servings</u>
A wonderful pie that is both filling and delicious.

Pie Crust
1 ½ cups (3 dl) hazelnuts
3 tbsp honey
1 tsp cardamom
½ tsp real vanilla powder

Filling
1 ½ cups (3 dl) cashews
¾ cup (1 ½ dl) water
½ avocado
2 tbsp honey
1 tsp vanilla powder

Topping:
8 plums
½ cup (1 dl) coconut flakes

Mix all of the ingredients for the crust in a food processor. Roll the dough out evenly and place in a springform pan. Let it chill in the refrigerator for 30 minutes.

Place the cashews, water, avocado, honey, and vanilla powder in a food processor and mix until it becomes a fluffy cream. Pour the cream into the pie crust. Cut the plums into wedges and arrange them on top. Decorate with coconut flakes.

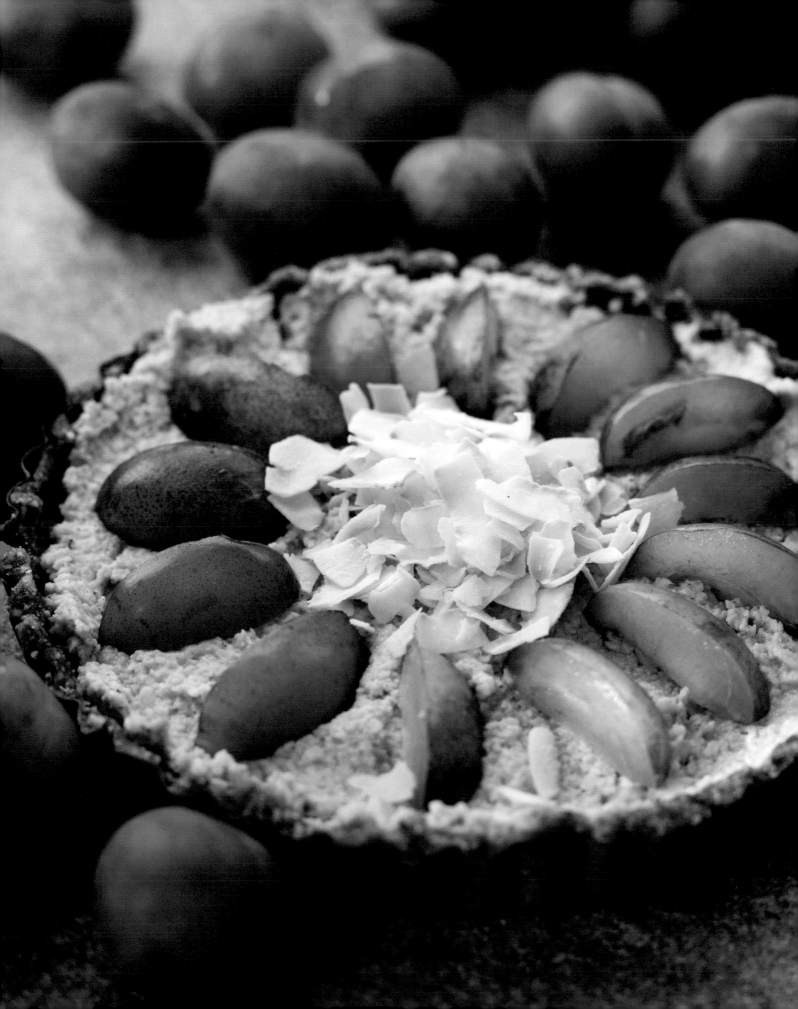

SAUCES & DIPS

Hummus with coriander and curry

1 batch
An amazingly tasty hummus.

2 cups (4 dl) canned chickpeas
2 garlic cloves
1 ½ tsp grated fresh ginger
½ cup (1 dl) chopped parsley
¼ cup (½ dl) chopped coriander
Juice of 1 lemon
½ tsp turmeric
½ tsp chili powder
1 tsp curry
¼ cup (½ dl) olive oil
Salt and black pepper

Mix all of the ingredients, except the oil, in a food processor. Pour the oil in slowly while the mixture is still blending. Continue to mix until it becomes an even spread. Season with salt and pepper.

Chunky olive tapenade

1 small batch
5 oz (½ jar) jarred pitted black olives
5 oz (½ jar) jarred pitted green olives
1 garlic clove
Fresh parsley
Lemon juice

Mix all of the ingredients in a food processor for a couple of seconds (the tapenade is supposed to be quite chunky, so do not overmix). Scoop the tapenade into a bowl and serve.

Hot bell pepper sauce

1 batch
This is the yummiest sauce and it goes with almost everything—just try it!

3.5 oz (100 g) shelled almonds
8–9 oz (250 g) canned roasted bell peppers
1 tbsp red wine vinegar
2 garlic cloves
1 tsp chili flakes
1 tsp salt
1 cup (2 dl) olive oil
½ cup (1 dl) sunflower seed oil

Mix all of the ingredients, except the oils, in a food processor. Add the oils slowly while the other ingredients are still blending. Mix until the sauce achieves an even consistency. Store the sauce in a cool place and stir before serving.

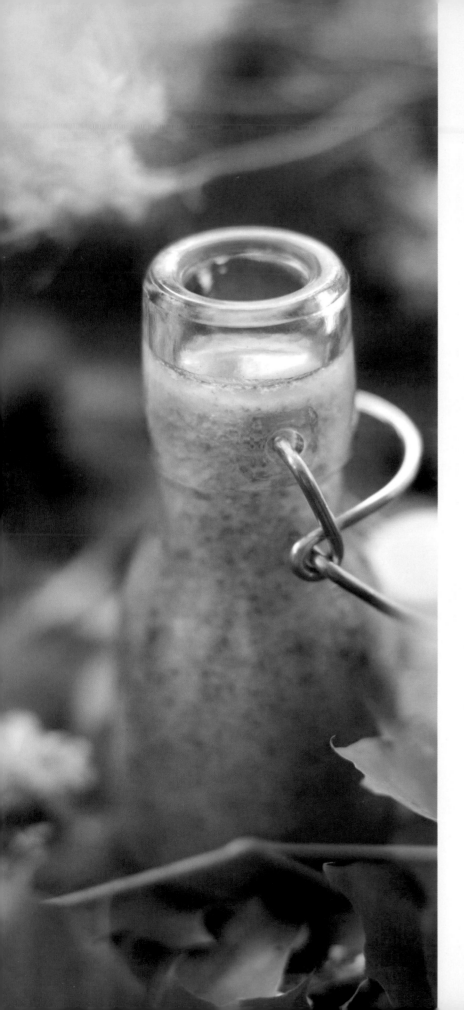

Mint pesto

<u>1 batch</u>
1 bunch mint leaves
¼ cup (½ dl) pine nuts
Juice of 1 lime
½ cup (1 dl) olive oil
Salt and black pepper

Mix the mint leaves, pine nuts, and lime juice in a food processor. Slowly pour the oil in the mixture and keep blending until it achieves an even consistency. Add salt and pepper according to taste.

Basil and dill pesto

<u>1 batch</u>
1 bunch basil
5 springs dill
1 garlic clove
Juice of ½ lemon
1.7 oz (50 g) pecorino cheese
½ cup (1 dl) olive oil
Salt and black pepper

Mix all of the ingredients, except the olive oil, in a food processor. Slowly pour the oil in the mixture and continue blending until it achieves an even consistency. Add salt and pepper according to taste. Store the pesto in a refrigerator.

Pea pesto

<u>1 batch</u>
3.5 oz (100 g) almonds
1 cup (2 dl) frozen peas
Juice of 1 lemon
1 garlic clove
1 cup (2 dl) olive oil
Salt and black pepper

Mix all of the ingredients, except the olive oil, in a food processor. Slowly pour the oil into the mixture and continue mixing until it achieves an even consistency. Add salt and pepper according to taste.

Red Pesto

<u>1 batch</u>
½ cup (1 dl) sundried tomatoes
2 garlic cloves
½ cup (1 dl) shelled almonds
½ cup (1 dl) grated parmesan cheese
¼–½ cup (½–1 dl) olive oil
Salt and black pepper

Mix all of the ingredients, except the olive oil, in a food processor. Slowly pour the oil into the mixture and continue mixing until it achieves an even consistency. Season with salt and pepper.

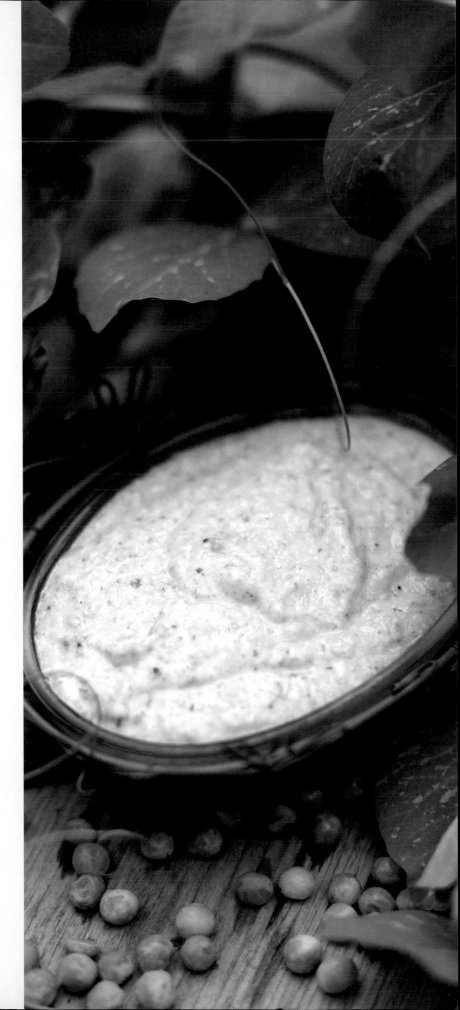

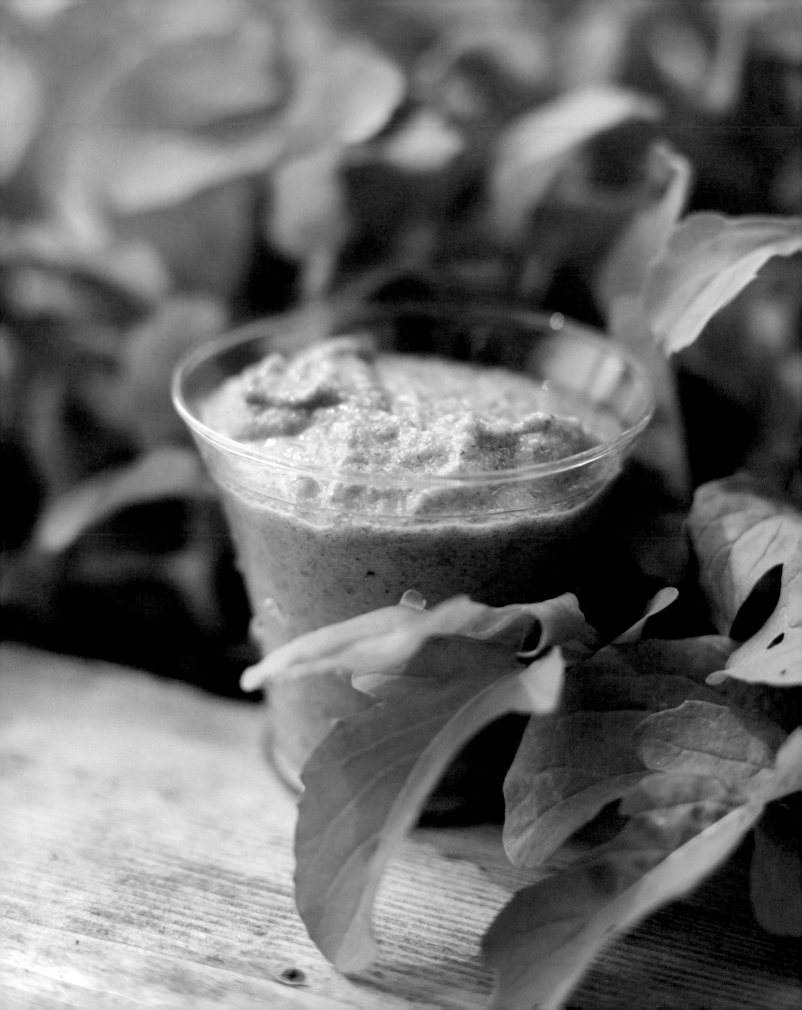

Arugula crème

<u>1 batch</u>
½ red onion
3.5 oz (100 g) arugula
½ cup (1 dl) walnuts
½ cup (1 dl) cashew nuts
1 garlic clove
¼ cup (½ dl) olive oil
½ cup (1 dl) canola oil
1 tsp honey
Salt and black pepper

Peel and chop the onion. Mix onion, arugula, walnuts, cashews, and garlic in a food processor. Slowly add the olive oil, canola oil, and honey while the mixture is still blending. Season with salt and pepper.

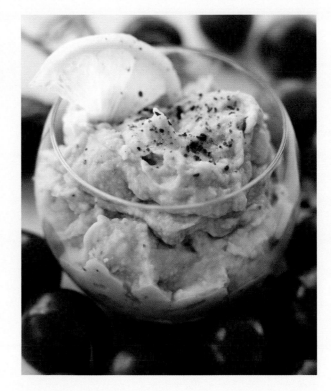

Mint guacamole

<u>1 batch</u>
2 ripe avocados
½–1 pressed garlic clove
1 bunch mint leaves
1 tbsp lemon juice
Salt and black pepper

Peel and cut up the avocados. Mix the avocado, garlic, and mint leaves in a food processor until the mixture becomes an even spread. Season with lemon juice, salt, and pepper.

Guacamole

<u>1 batch</u>
½ red onion
1 ripe tomato
2 ripe avocados
½–1 pressed garlic clove
1 tbsp lemon juice
1–2 pinches cayenne
Salt and black pepper

Peel and chop the onion, tomatoes, and avocados. Place in a food processor with the garlic. Mix until even and season with lemon juice, cayenne, salt, and pepper.

Orange and mint dressing

<u>1 batch</u>
Goes great with all kinds of salads.

Juice of 2 oranges
½ cup (1 dl) olive oil
2 tbsp white wine vinegar
½ cup (1 dl) mint leaves
Salt and black pepper

Mix all of the ingredients in a food processor for a few minutes. Pour the dressing in a glass bottle or other closed container. Store in the refrigerator.

Asian dipping sauce

<u>1 batch</u>
1–2 tbsp rice vinegar
1 tbsp light soy sauce
½ tsp sesame oil
2 tbsp canola oil
2 tbsp chopped coriander
½ tsp muscovado sugar
½ tsp sambal oelek (chili paste)
1 tbsp water

Mix all ingredients together in a bowl and place in the fridge.

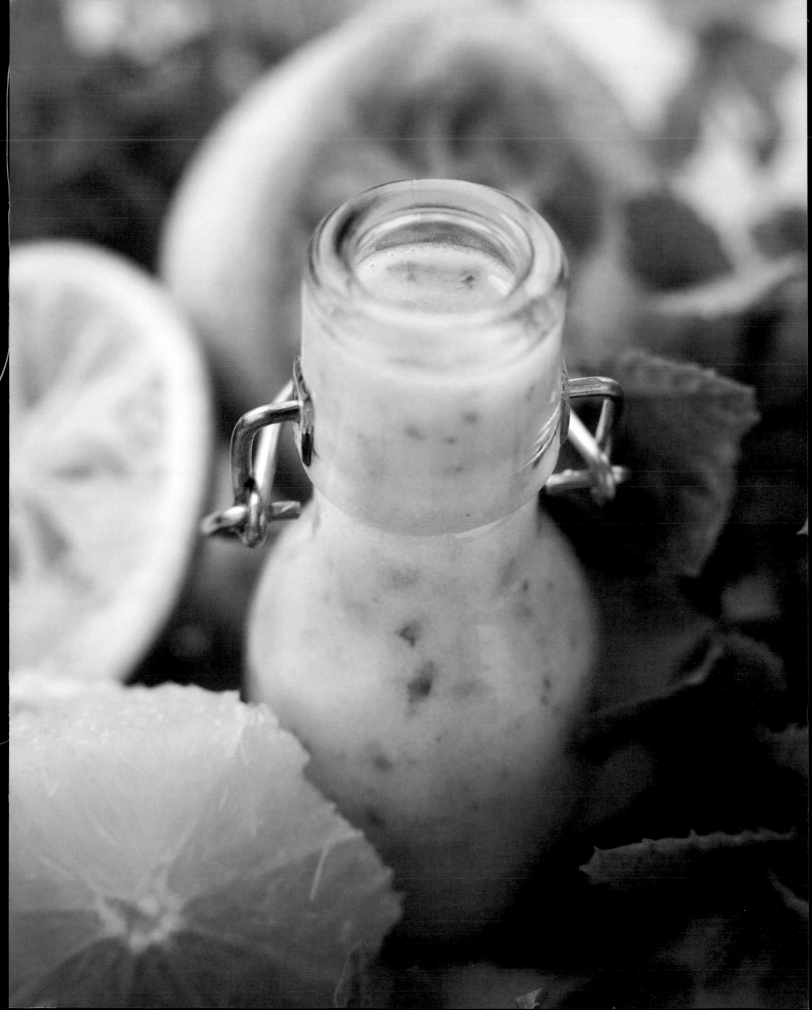

RECIPE INDEX